Innovative Medical Devices

By involving China and international experts in medical devices and allied technologies, the book series covers both original research and practical approaches to device innovation and aims to be served as an important reference to researchers and developers in medical devices and related fields. The book series include 7 topics, which are strategic frontiers, medical imaging, in vitro diagnosis, advanced therapeutics, medical rehabilitation, health promotion and biomedical materials.

The book series reflects the latest developments in the fields and is suitable for senior undergraduates, postgraduates, managers, and research and development engineers in medical devices companies and regulatory bodies, as well as medical students. The book series is also suitable for training in related topics.

Yao Guo • Giulio Dagnino
Guang-Zhong Yang

Medical Robotics

History, Challenges, and Future Directions

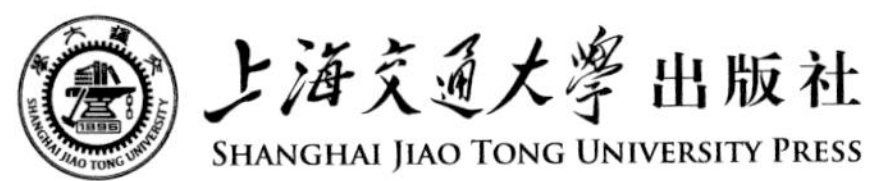

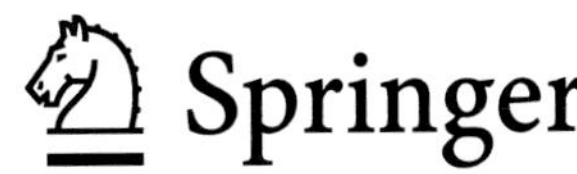

Yao Guo
Institute of Medical Robotics
Shanghai Jiao Tong University
Shanghai, China

Guang-Zhong Yang
Institute of Medical Robotics
Shanghai Jiao Tong University
Shanghai, China

Giulio Dagnino
Robotics and Mechatronics
University of Twente
Enschede, Overijssel, The Netherlands

ISSN 2731-7730 ISSN 2731-7749 (electronic)
Innovative Medical Devices

ISBN 978-981-99-7319-4 ISBN 978-981-99-7317-0 (eBook)
https://doi.org/10.1007/978-981-99-7317-0

Jointly published with Shanghai Jiao Tong University Press
The print edition is not for sale in China (Mainland). Customers from China (Mainland) please order the print book from: Shanghai Jiao Tong University Press.

This Springer imprint is published by the registered company Springer Nature Singapore Pte Ltd.
The registered company address is: 152 Beach Road, #21-01/04 Gateway East, Singapore 189721, Singapore

Paper in this product is recyclable.

Preface

Medical robotics for surgery, personalized rehabilitation, hospital automation, and high-throughput screening represents an important area of growth globally. Driven by increasing clinical emphases on improved surveillance and earlier diagnosis, it is moving into an era of precision intervention, demanding improved quality, minimally invasive access, and an unprecedented level of accuracy. The commercial success of the early-generation medical robots has inspired an ever-increasing number of platforms from both commercial and research organizations, resulting in more agile and intelligent systems. This book looks back through the last decades at how medical robotics has evolved into a major area of innovation and development involving integrated multidisciplinary collaborative effort. With improved safety, efficacy, and reduced costs, robotic platforms will soon approach a tipping point, moving beyond early adopters to become mainstream clinical practice, also defining the future of smart hospitals and home-based patient care.

This book is intended as an introductory literature by outlining the global trends and new research directions in medical robotics, highlighting associated technical, commercial, regulatory, and economic challenges. In particular, this book focuses on three areas of medical robotics: (1) robotic surgery (Chaps. 2 and 3), (2) rehabilitation robotics (Chaps. 4 and 5), and (3) hospital automation (Chap. 6). For each subject area, important clinical needs and technical aspects are discussed, focusing on practical systems and research publications that have contributed to key advances in medical robotics in recent years. Open challenges and future opportunities are identified and discussed in Chap. 7.

Shanghai, China — Yao Guo
Enschede, Overijssel, The Netherlands — Giulio Dagnino
Shanghai, China — Guang-Zhong Yang
February 2023

Acknowledgments

We would like to thank our colleagues at the Institute of Medical Robotics, Shanghai Jiao Tong University, and the Robotics and Mechatronics group, University of Twente, for their contribution during the preparation of this book. In particular, we would like to thank Prof Weidong Chen, Dr Dennis Kundrat, Mr Xiao Gu, and Ms Rui Gu for their help with contributing materials used in this book. Our special thanks go to Ms Ziyi Zhang for her beautiful and meticulous graphical illustrations specially designed for us.

We would also like to thank Dr Christina Flann at the University of Twente for the proofreading service, and the editorial staff of Shanghai Jiao Tong University Press and Springer in helping with the editorial matters.

Yao Guo, Giulio Dagnino, and Guang-Zhong Yang

Contents

Introduction 1

Contents

"*Medical robotics is a rapidly advancing area of development, spearheading the evolution of precision medicine, personalized rehabilitation, and hospital automation. The commercial success of the early-generation medical robotic systems has inspired an ever-increasing number of platforms from both commercial and research organizations, resulting in smaller, safer, and smarter devices for general clinical use.*" Medical robots include surgical robotics, rehabilitation and assistive robotics, and hospital automation robotics, as shown in Fig. 1.1. This book looks back through the last decades at how medical robotics has evolved into a major area of innovation and development. With improved safety, efficacy, and reduced costs, robotic platforms will soon approach a tipping point, moving beyond early adopters to become part of the mainstream clinical practice, defining the future of smart hospitals and home-based patient care. These platforms will also have a greater focus on early intervention and quality of life after treatment. This book outlines the global trends and new research directions of medical robotics, highlighting associated technical, commercial, regulatory, and economic challenges.

Y. Guo et al., *Medical Robotics*, Innovative Medical Devices,
https://doi.org/10.1007/978-981-99-7317-0_1

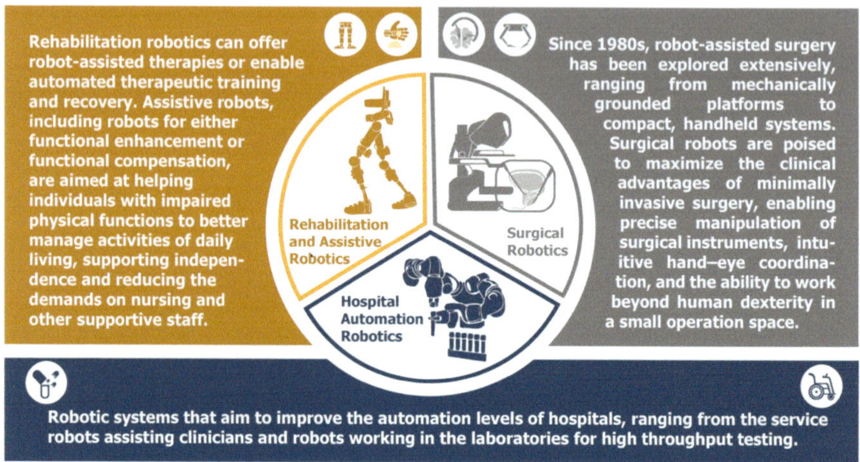

Fig. 1.1 Taxonomy of medical robotics. Medical robotics can be categorized into surgical robotics, rehabilitation and assistive robotics, and hospital automation robotics

1.1 Rise of Surgical Robotics

Since the end of the 1960s, when Driller and Neumann published the very first medical robot-related paper [1], the field of medical robotics has been in constant development. However, it was only in the mid-1980s that the concept of Health and Service Robotics was introduced, when the United States Congress was urged to support "*innovative research in functional rehabilitation of cognitive capabilities, speech, mobility, and manipulation*." During that period, robots in medicine were considered mainly as rehabilitation devices and nursing assistants [2]. In 1985, a conventional industrial robot, the Puma 200 (Unimation Inc., Danbury, CT) [3], was experimentally employed in a surgical procedure of needle insertion, demonstrating the first example of a surgical robot in history. Since then, an ever-increasing number of platforms from both commercial and research organizations have been developed and successfully used in a wide range of surgical specializations, such as neurosurgery, *Ear-Nose-Throat* (ENT), orthopedics, laparoscopy, and endoluminal intervention [2, 4–12].

Figure 1.2 shows the timeline of surgical robots, showing some of the platforms that have marked the last 30 years of surgical robotics development. The first generation of surgical robots relates to stereotaxic interventions in neurosurgery and orthopedics. For example, the Neuromate system (Renishaw, New Mills, UK) allows accurate neurological tool positioning procedures [14] (e.g., for biopsy, neuroendoscopy, and electrode implantation) using a robotic tool handler. ROBODOC (Curexo Technology, Fremont, CA) was the first surgical robotic system for orthopedics (i.e., hip replacement) that reached the market in 1994 [15].

The 1990s signified a move from stereotaxic robotic systems to the second-generation surgical robots, i.e., rigid yet dexterous robots for *Minimally Invasive Surgery* (MIS). The ZEUS platform (Computer Motion, Goleta, USA) [16] is the

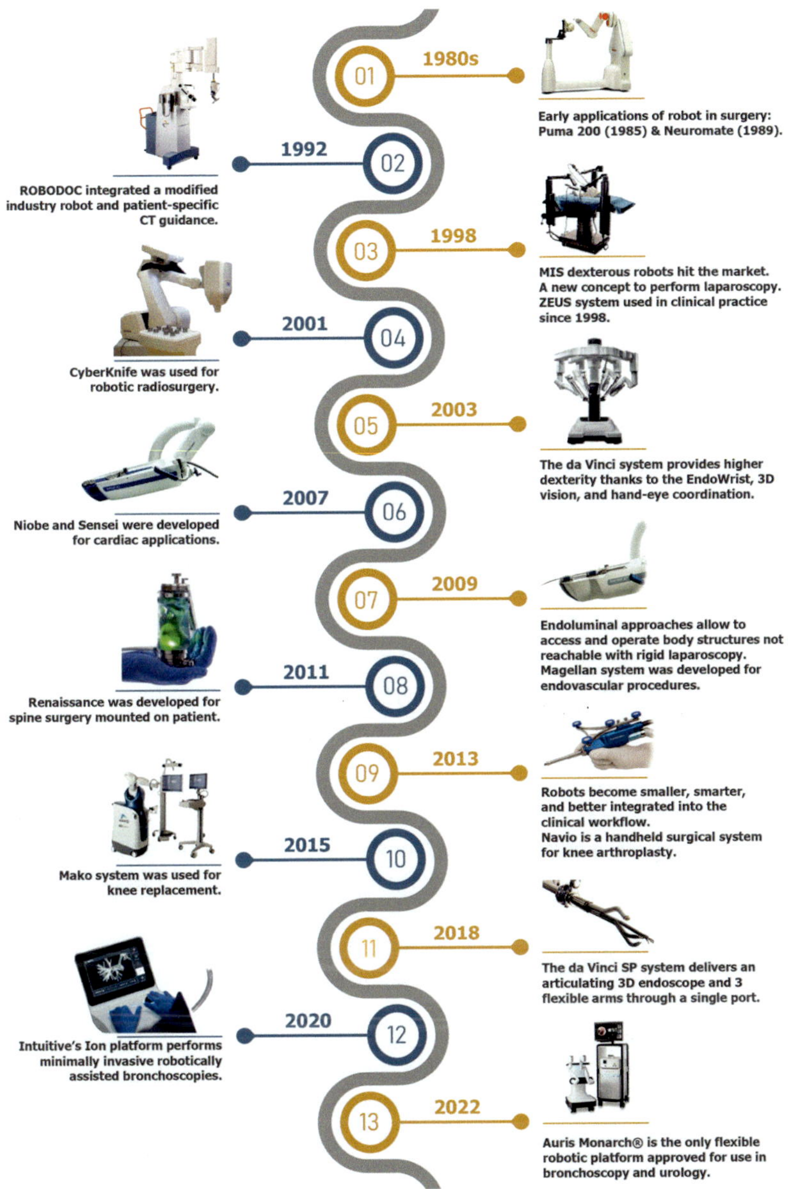

Fig. 1.2 Timeline of surgical robots. Since the first application of a robot in surgery in 1985, a growing number of robotic surgical platforms have been developed and applied to several clinical specializations. From bulky industrial arms adapted to be used in clinical applications—typical of the infancy of robotic surgery—robotic platforms have been bespoke designed to facilitate clinical usability and have become smaller and smarter. This figure reports key milestones in robotics surgery (only commercial platforms) over the last 40 years. Neuromate, Renishaw, © 2023; ROBODOC (CC BY 4.0); ZEUS/AESOP, © Computer Motion; CyberKnife, (CC BY 2.0); da Vinci/da Vinci SP/Ion, Intuitive Surgical Inc., © 2023; Sensei and Niobe (adapted with Springer Nature permission from [13]); Mazor Robotics Renaissance, Mazor Robotics; Navio, Smith & Nephew, © 2023; Mako, Stryker, © 2023; Monarch, Johnson & Johnson MedTech, © 2023

first platform developed for laparoscopy in 1998. It presents several robotic arms that operate inside the patient controlled by the surgeon sitting on a remote console. ZEUS was first applied to cardio-surgery and became famous in 2001 for the trans-oceanic cholecystectomy successfully performed by Marescaux and colleagues [17]. A patient in Strasbourg, France, had her gall bladder removed using ZEUS and was teleoperated by surgeons in New York. The da Vinci system (Intuitive Surgical, Sunnyvale, USA)—now likely the most famous commercial surgical robot world-wide—replaced ZEUS in 2003. The da Vinci systems feature immersive 3D visualization of the surgical scene via a remote console that allows the teleoperation of the laparoscopic instruments. Such configuration allows hand–eye coordination while providing stereo-vision of the surgical field, something not possible in standard laparoscopy. Intuitive Surgical developed many versions of the da Vinci system (e.g., the multi-arm version da Vinci Xi, and the single port version da Vinci SP), which have been used in many clinical applications such as cardiosurgery, colorectal surgery, prostatectomy, and many others [18].

The evolution of surgical robots toward smaller and smarter devices continues in the first decade of this millennium, allowing robots to be used in transluminal or endoluminal procedures. The third generation of surgical robots, i.e., flexible robots for MIS, includes small and steerable devices, such as robotic catheters or snake-like robots, which can access and operate in constrained regions of the human body not previously reachable with rigid laparoscopy. Endovascular procedures can be executed under robotic assistance, using, for example, the two major commercial platforms developed by Hansen Medical (acquired by Auris Health Inc., Redwood City, USA): the Sensei X2 (for *electrophysiological* (EP) procedures) and the Magellan (for endovascular applications) [19, 20]. The i-Snake developed by Yang and his colleagues [21], a snake-like system, allows exploration of a large area of the anatomy through *Natural Orifice Transluminal Endoscopic Surgery* (NOTES) without requiring laparoscopic-style external manipulation, and it has full retroflection capabilities [22].

Concentric tube robots [5] address the limitations of catheter robots by providing higher stiffness while maintaining the required steerability. They are created by a number of pre-curved interconnected elastic tubes that steer when translated and rotated with respect to one another. Since 2005, this technology has become attractive for robot-assisted surgical applications thanks to the pioneering work of Sears & Dupont [23], Webster [24], and Furusho et al. [25], and further evolved to the current stage thanks to technical advances in design [26], control [27], sensing [28], and image guidance [29]. For example, the Monarch platform (Auris Health Inc., Redwood City, USA) integrates robotics and enhanced navigation (3D imaging and sensing) for bronchoscopy applications and received *Food and Drug Administration* (FDA) approval in April 2018. Untethered micro-surgical devices, such as wireless capsules for endoscopy and micro- and nano-robots, are the fourth generation of surgical robots [30]. Endoscopy capsules were introduced in the early 2000s and have evolved thanks to the research of several groups worldwide [31–33], becoming an alternative to traditional endoscopy of the *gastrointestinal* (GI) tract [31–34].

1.2 Popularity of Rehabilitation and Assistive Robotics

The aging population is imposing unprecedented challenges on chronic disease and health management since the elderly are at high risk of motor weakness, cardiovascular diseases, and neurological and musculoskeletal disorders, leading to a high potential of impaired cognitive and physical functions [35]. For instance, stroke has become the leading cardiovascular disease that causes death and disability worldwide. Most patients who survive stroke encounter reduced capability of upper-limb movement, hand manipulation, or even walking [36]. Additionally, neurodegenerative diseases are also affecting a large population in the world, where patients demonstrate diverse motor symptoms and cognitive impairment [37], bringing an increasing burden of personal care in daily life. Hence, there is a pressing need for patients to receive long-term rehabilitation training in hospitals or in home-based environments, recovering patients' functionalities of neurological to musculoskeletal systems progressively. For those with disabilities or motor weakness, personal assistance and functional augmentation are of paramount importance in aiding patients to complete *Activities of Daily Living* (ADL).

Commonly, rehabilitation training is guided by professional therapists at either hospitals or rehabilitation centers, including physical therapy, occupational therapy, speech-language therapy, or psychotherapy. However, such training requires labor-intensive repeated work provided by the therapists. Disabled patients or people with impaired physical functions frequently need around-the-clock assistance from two to three caregivers or to complete ADL. However, compared to the high demand of patients requiring rehabilitation training or personal assistance, the number of therapists or caregivers is far from sufficient.

To fulfill such demands in healthcare, the development of rehabilitation and assistive robots has been actively pursued in the past decades. In particular, robotic systems are aimed at either assisting/empowering individuals to complete ADL tasks or improving the recovery of individuals' physical/cognitive functioning through automatic therapeutic training [38–41]. Rehabilitation and assistive robotics is a multidisciplinary field involving robotics, bioinformatics, anatomy, mechanical engineering, material science, control theory, and *Human–Robot Interaction* (HRI). As robots are advantageous in providing long-term and repeated movement, rehabilitation robots can offer automatic therapeutic training like therapists [38]. To provide either functional augmentation (e.g., exoskeleton) or functional compensation (e.g., prosthesis and intelligent wheelchair), a number of assistive robots have been developed for assisting with different ADL tasks, helping patients to better manage ADL or supporting independence and reducing the demands for nursing or other supportive staff [39, 40, 42]. As such, robots are typically connected to or collaborate closely with patients. Extensive research effort has been gained on the development of robots with soft and dexterous mechanical structure as well as natural and intelligent HRI mechanisms.

Figure 1.3 gives an overview of the development history and current state of rehabilitation and assistive robots. As there exist numerous robots for

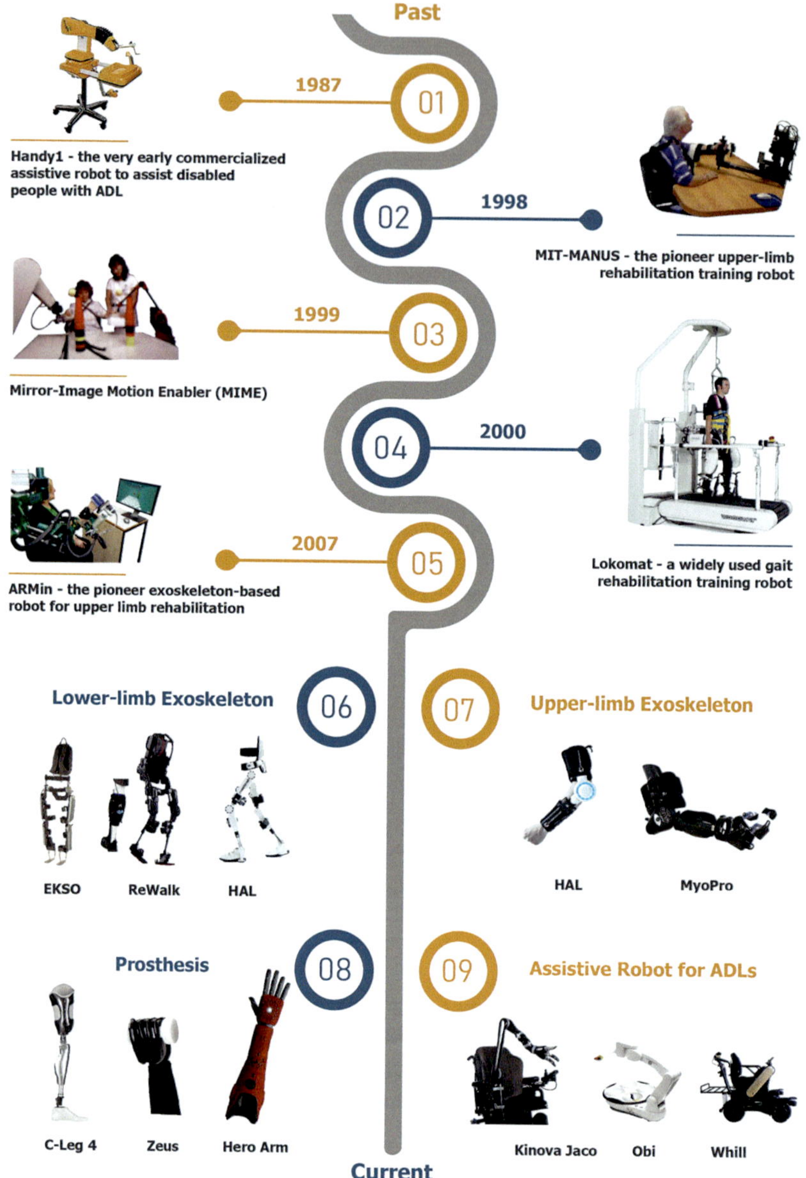

Fig. 1.3 Research states of rehabilitation and assistive robots: from past to current state of the art. With the advancement in multidisciplinary technologies, recent research attention has been shifted from large/grounded systems to lightweight/wearable ones. Handy 1 (adapted with Springer Nature permission from [43]); MIT-MANUS (adapted with Taylor & Francis permission from [44]); MIME (adapted from [45] (CC BY 4.0)); Lokomat (adapted from [46] (CC BY 4.0)); ARMin (adapted from [47] (CC BY 4.0)); EKSO, Ekso Bionics, © 2022; ReWalk, ReWalk Robotics Inc., © 2023; HAL, Copyright by CYBERDYNE Inc.; MyoPro, Myomo, © 2023; C-Leg4, Copyright by Ottobock; Zeus, Aether Biomedical, © 2023; Hero Arm, Open Bionics, © 2022; Kinova Jaco, Kinova Inc., © 2023; Obi, Obi, © 2023; Whill, WHILL Inc., © 2015–2023

rehabilitation training and personal assistance, here we only summarize several landmark robots and those that have been approved for clinical use. The very early commercialized assistive robot, namely Handy1, was developed by Mike Topping in 1987. Handy1 is a robotic system that is capable of assisting the most severely disabled people with several ADL tasks, such as eating, drinking, washing, teeth cleaning, and shaving [43]. The MIT-MANUS robot, developed in the 1990s, was the pioneer upper-limb rehabilitation training robot that achieved successful commercial applications during the past decades [48]. This end-effector-based robotic system is able to guide the movement of a subject's upper limb while playing interactive games. In 1999, a *Mirror-Image Motion Enabler* (MIME) was developed by Stanford University, using a Puma 560 robotic arm to guide the 3 *Degree of Freedom* (DoF) motion of the affected side by reproducing the movement of the patient's healthy side [45]. Due to the motion compensation and limited *Range of Motion* (RoM) induced by end-effector-based robotic systems, researchers shifted their attention to developing grounded exoskeletons for rehabilitation. Among numerous grounded systems, ARMin was a pioneer exoskeleton-based robot for upper-limb rehabilitation [49], which could provide either passive or active therapeutic training. For lower-limb rehabilitation, a widely used gait rehabilitation training robot, namely Lokomat, was developed by Hocoma (Hocoma, Volketswil, Switzerland) in 2000. The Lokomat is a robotic treadmill-based gait training system, where the individuals are suspended and their legs are attached to a robotic exoskeleton [50].

With the rapid progress in electronics, materials, *Artificial Intelligence* (AI), and robotics, recent rehabilitation and assistive robots have gained popularity in developing lightweight and wearable systems. Most of these systems are embedded with advanced robot control and intelligent HRI techniques. [51, 52] In addition to end-effector-based and grounded exoskeleton systems [45, 48–50], wearable upper-limb and lower-limb exoskeletons [53, 54] have been successfully commercialized, providing rehabilitation training and assistance for individuals recovering from stroke or spinal cord injury. ReWalk (ReWalk Robotics Inc., Marlborough, US) was the first wearable lower-limb exoskeleton that got FDA approval [53] (hospital use in 2011 and public use in 2014). EKSO (Ekso Bionics, Berkeley, US), formerly known as *Human Universal Load Carrier* (HULC) [54], was the first wearable exoskeleton cleared by the FDA for use with stroke patients. *Hybrid Assistive Limb* (HAL), developed by CYBERDYNE (CYBERDYNE Inc., Tsukuba, Japan), was the first wearable cyborg for both upper and lower limbs [55]. Additionally, intelligent prostheses incorporating the *Human–Machine Interface* (HMI) can help amputees perform daily tasks, where diverse interfaces with bidirectional links can be established between motor and sensory functions. Meanwhile, various types of assistive robots have become practical in different scenarios, empowering individuals' capability or assisting them to better complete ADL. For instance, assistant robotic arms are able to grasp objects for users or help them finish dining. Intelligent wheelchairs can help disabled people navigate through the environment automatically.

1.3 Emergence of Hospital Automation Robotics

In addition to medical robots that are directly used in the clinical treatment and diagnosis during surgery, as well as rehabilitation training and personal assistance in daily life, another significant category lies in automation robots that aim to improve the level of automation in hospitals. Specifically, the scenarios for hospital automation robots can be classified into five categories: (1) robotics for hospital logistics; (2) pharmacy and drug management; (3) patient transfer and care; (4) high throughput lab automation; and (5) robots for diagnosis and imaging, as illustrated in Fig. 1.4.

In recent years, different service robot systems have emerged in hospitals to help with logistic and routine tasks, including reception, disinfection, inventory management, and in-hospital delivery. For instance, logistic robots can automatically navigate through the complicated environment in the hospital, dispensing or collecting medical supplies or wastes. Nowadays, more and more robots with speech interaction and interactive interfaces can serve as receptionists, providing guidance for those patients who need help. Especially during the spread of *Coronavirus Disease 2019* (COVID-19), such robots for hospital logistics demonstrated prominent potential in combating infectious diseases [57, 58], preventing medical staff from exposure to potential risks. In addition, disinfection robots have become widely available during the fight against COVID-19 [59]. Robotic disinfection embraces multiple approaches, but the most commonly used ones use *Ultraviolet* (UV) light to destroy microorganisms. A recent study demonstrated the effectiveness of UV treatment against three different viruses, including SARS-CoV-1 [60].

Pharmacy and drug management is labor-intensive and requires meticulous attention in hospitals, where robotic systems can significantly improve the efficiency, accuracy, and safety of the workflow in the pharmacy department [61]. These robots aim to help medical staff reduce labor-intensive and repeated tasks (e.g., picking and placing drugs in bins) and allow them to focus on their area of expertise. Currently, robotic arms are widely used for drug management and dispensing, which can provide dexterous manipulation and grasping like human beings [62]. Moreover, robotic systems can help reduce the potential contamination induced by human workers, enabling zero-touch and zero-error pharmacy automation. Robots can also be used for drug blending with high speed, such as intravenous drugs and anti-tumor chemotherapy drugs.

Another significant role of hospital automation robotics is for nursing purposes. These robots can provide oversight not only in inpatient wards but also in the Intensive Care Unit (ICU), providing 24/7 monitoring and assistance for patients with needs. In particular, for paraplegic patients or people with motor weakness, nursing and transfer robots have emerged to provide support for patients to complete sit-to-stand/stand-to-sit or transfer them from one place to another, which can significantly save the effort of caregivers [63]. In addition, some service robots are developed to cooperate with surgeons, assisting in surgery in the operation room [64]. It should be emphasized that most transfer robots (e.g., intelligent wheelchairs) are built upon mobile platforms. By integrating advanced sensing [e.g., computer vision, *Light Detection and Ranging* (LIDAR)] technologies], localization

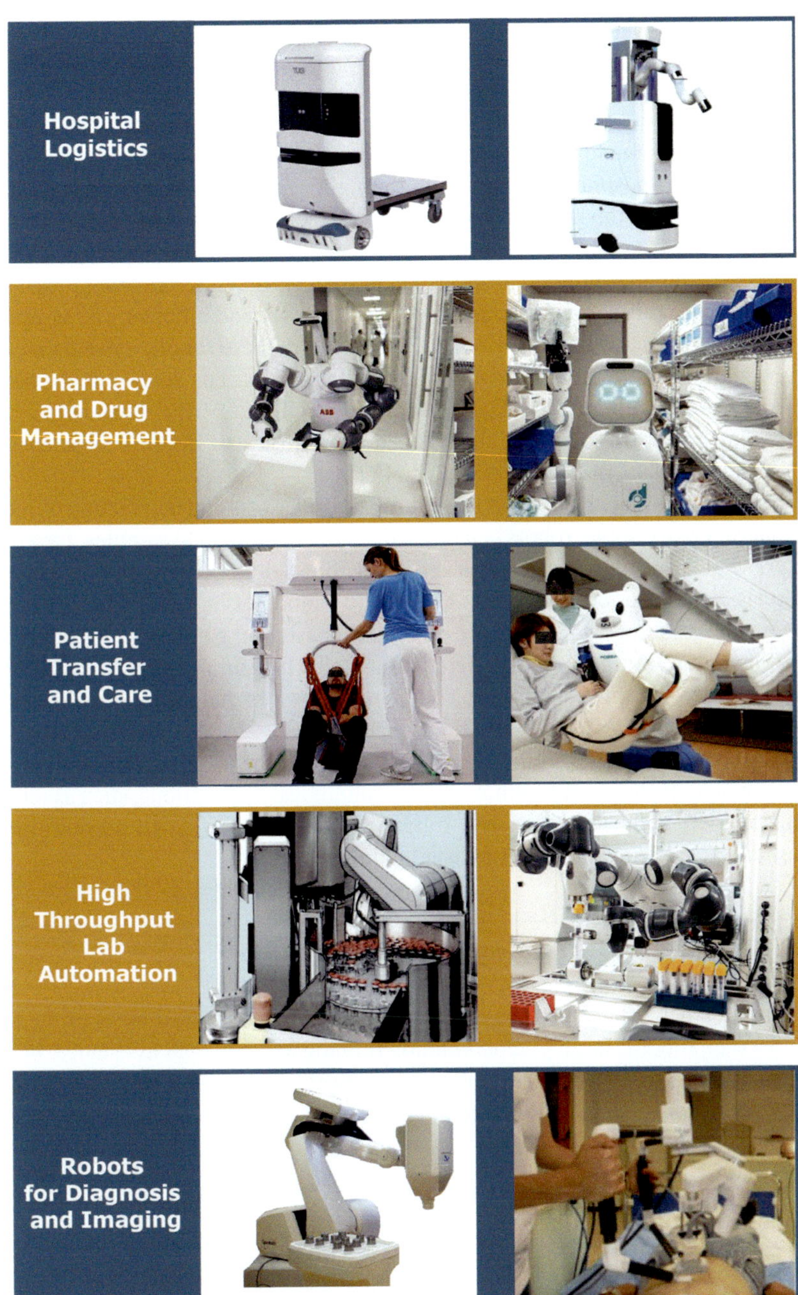

Fig. 1.4 Main categories of available hospital automation robots. The figure shows the hospital automation robots that are working for hospital logistics (TUG, Aethon © 2018; Guardian II, Guangdong Jaten Robot & Automation Co., Ltd., © 2022), drug management (YuMi, ABB, © 2023; Moxi, Diligent Robotics Inc., © 2023), patient transfer and care (PTR, Copyright © PTR Robots; Robear, Copyright © RIKEN, Japan), high throughput lab automation (Pharma, DSG Robotics, © 2017–2020 by Netech; YuMi, ABB, © 2023), and diagnosis and imaging (CyberKnife, Wikimedia Commons (CC BY 2.0); MELODY, adapted from [56], CC BY 4.0)

and navigation in the cluttered hospital environment can be achieved automatically. Meanwhile, intelligent robots are able to recognize human targets or objects of interest, allowing the completion of more complicated tasks (e.g., object manipulation and patient transfer). Robots with a single arm or bimanual arms can perform various dexterous manipulations or cooperate with human workers.

In addition to hospital logistics, high throughput testing robots play significant roles in improving the automation levels of the laboratories [65], which include robotic platforms used for automated liquid handling, automated synthesis, DNA/RNA sequencing, in vitro diagnosis, and data analysis and interpretation [66]. With the help of high throughput testing robots, the accuracy and efficiency of assay and synthesis can be significantly guaranteed. In addition, these robotic systems used in single-cell transcriptomics, proteomics, and metabolomics can accelerate the development of precision medicine. For instance, during the COVID-19 pandemic, high throughput testing robots have shown their capabilities to improve efficiency in nucleic acid test and vaccine development [57].

Finally, robots can also help in facilitating the diagnosis and acquisition of medical images. For example, robots can be used to collect biological samples, for *Point-of-Care* (PoC) diagnosis, in ICUs, and even within radiology departments both for diagnosis and treatment purposes. Diagnostic blood testing and oro- and naso-pharyngeal swabbing can be performed by a robot during pandemics to reduce the risk of infection for the operators. Telerobots can be helpful in applications where a remote doctor takes all the physiological parameters and diagnoses a disease using audiovisual aids. ICU robots can be used to provide access to off-site patients, supervising physicians, and other specialists, making otherwise very difficult procedures possible. Robots can be employed in radiological applications, such as remote acquisition of medical images and robot-assisted therapies, such as performing ultrasound acquisition and robot-assisted radiotherapy.

1.4 Emerging Technologies and Challenges

The common denominator in the evolution of the aforementioned areas of medical robotics (i.e., robotic surgery, rehabilitation training and personal assistance, hospital automation) is the general evolution of medical technologies, which eventually brought together robotics, AI, imaging, and sensing.

1.4.1 Robotic Surgery

For surgical robotics, this process started long ago with the first endoscope (Bozzini, 1806), followed by the discovery of X-rays (Roentgen, 1895). A few years later, *Computer Tomography* (CT) and *Magnetic Resonance Imaging* (MRI) allowed us to acquire and visualize 3D data of the anatomy, paving the way to improved pre-operative planning and the intra-operative navigation of clinical procedures thanks to computer assistance. The so-called *Computer Assisted Intervention* (CAI) was born, and its main goal was to assist clinicians to perform better both in terms of diagnosis and treatment of diseases. CAI is used in combination with surgical robots to connect patient-specific data with precision technology able to sense and interact with the human body. In this sense, the integration of sensing and imaging with robotics is fundamental not only to support clinical decisions but to enable autonomous or semiautonomous navigation features.

Surgical robots are becoming smaller following the advances in precision manufacturing, microfabrication, and materials. Micro-robots can navigate the human body to perform treatment and diagnosis of pathologies. In the future, micro- and nano-robots will be able to reach target cells, recognize the pathology, and attack it locally while preserving the healthy tissues [2]. This will be possible thanks to advances in the areas of microfabrication, power optimization, imaging, and sensing technologies [4].

Artificial Intelligence (AI) and machine learning will make robots smarter and able to interact with the clinical environment with increased levels of autonomy [67]. This will necessarily grow hand-in-hand with enhanced navigation and mapping techniques so that robots will be able to understand the clinical procedure and cooperate with the clinician to achieve one or more clinical tasks, or even make decisions in full autonomy [68]. According to Yang et al. [69], "the grand challenge for robotic navigation is to develop systems able to effectively learn from unmapped/unknown environments and dynamically adapt to them, similar to how human perception works. Robotic navigation requires semantic understanding and representation of scenes and active interactions."

Another key point is the interaction between users and robots (i.e., HRI). HRI aims to establish uni- or bi-directional communication/interaction between robotic systems and humans, including haptic feedback, brain–machine interfaces, gestures, and eye or vocal control [70]. Physical interfaces, currently the most commonly used, are generally master controllers that the user manipulates to operate a remote surgical robot and accomplish tasks such as tissue manipulation or tool handling [71]. Those basic approaches can be combined with *Learning from Demonstration* (LfD) of human experts to gain autonomy for task execution [72]. Designs of HRI are governed by task-specific requirements, ergonomics, and guidelines, as summarized in Adamides et al. [73], especially when used for clinical applications where easiness of use and clinical acceptance are of paramount importance.

1.4.2 Robots for Cognitive Rehabilitation and Social Assistance

In the past decades, there has been extensive attention paid to the development of rehabilitation and assistive robots focusing on therapeutic training or personal assistance of human physical functions. However, the number of patients encountering neurological disorders [e.g., *Alzheimer's Disease* (AD), *Parkinson's Disease* (PD), and *Autism Spectrum Disorders* (ASD)] has dramatically increased recently. These patients have demonstrated various types of impairment in memory, learning ability, communication, and social interaction, thus requiring extensive effort in care and companionship. Therefore, it is of paramount significance in the development of cognition rehabilitation and socially assistive robots [74].

Due to the patients' behavioral and cognitive abnormalities, one of the prerequisites of such robots is to establish intelligent and reliable HRI to understand their behavior and cognition [51, 75]. For instance, human posture and action could indicate their motion intention, while facial expression and eye movement imply their emotions and mental states. In addition, analysis of their brain activities plays a significant role in exploring the underlying mechanism between patients' behavior and cognition. To achieve this, multimodal sensing techniques along with dedicated machine learning algorithms are critical steps [76].

Commonly, the intervention provided by specialists is the main treatment for patients with cognitive impairment. As disparity exists among patients and there are differences in their behaviors, another significant challenge is to establish personalized intervention, including cognition assessment, treatment plan development, and social interaction [77]. Hence, there remain great opportunities to develop personalized artificial intelligent algorithms and HRI mechanisms.

Another important topic within cognitive rehabilitation and socially assistive robots is delivering effective feedback to patients, such as facial expression, pronunciation and intonation, eye contact, and body language [78]. Along this line, robots can gain the trust of users, which could facilitate effective social interaction between patients and robots. Moreover, ethics and regulations are very important in the development of such robots, as they may live/work with patients in their homes. Moreover, data storage, privacy, and encryption are also significant issues that need to be considered.

1.4.3 Robots for the Future of Smart Hospitals

Figure 1.5 points out several key characteristics of the future of smart hospitals. First of all, it is essential to push the less-complex medical support out of major hospitals and into a home-based environment and local community. Hence, a hierarchical healthcare delivery system could be established, including in-home care, polyclinics, community hospitals, and super hospitals. The advancement of pervasive sensing and telepresence robots enables the deployment of better and cheaper diagnostics and monitoring in the home. For most patients, polyclinics and community hospitals with walk-in distance are able to provide face-to-face care, where standard medical treatment and healthcare support could be given. For those who want to receive high-quality and all-round healthcare service, super hospitals are able to provide personalized medicine through long-term monitoring of multimodal healthcare data.

As one of the cutting-edge technologies, medical robotics has been extensively applied to solve problems in clinical treatment, and the problems found in clinical practice are fed back to indicate the direction of research focus, so as to achieve a closed loop of technological innovation and clinical translation. Therefore, smart

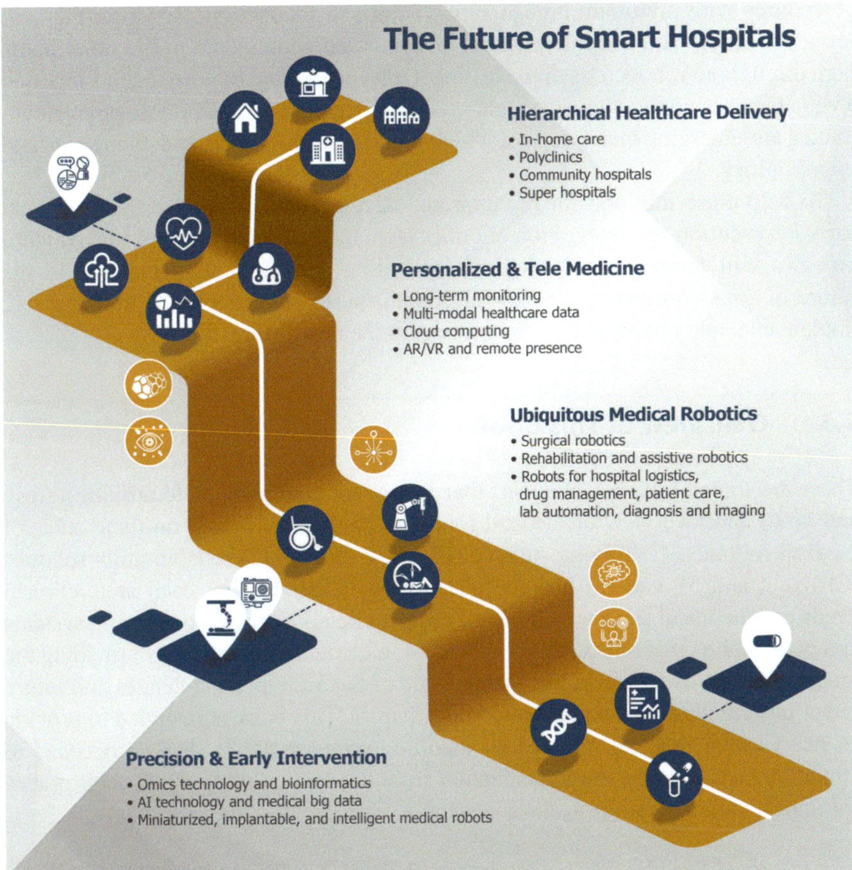

Fig. 1.5 A prospect of the future smart hospitals

super hospitals with levels of automation will become prevalent in the near future [4]. Rather than robot-assisted surgery and rehabilitation, increasing attention has been gained on building robotics systems that engage in hospital logistics, pharmacy, drug management, and patient transfer and care. The development of future service robots could focus on the integration of multiple intelligent systems to form a complete and automated workflow in hospitals. Each robot is not only responsible for a specific task but can cooperate with other robots to achieve more complicated tasks. In addition, future service robots in a smart hospital should be multi-functional, which means that they can undertake different tasks automatically, collaborating with human workers in a safe and seamless manner. Robots for diagnosis and imaging will be more widely used in routine clinical practice. This will require advances in imaging and sensing technologies to guarantee safe and reliable applications of robotic devices to perform diagnoses on patients. Autonomy will play a key role in the advances of such systems to perform diagnostic and treatment procedures with minimum human supervision and interaction. However, this will introduce safety and ethical concerns that must be addressed. On the other hand, high throughput robots for sample testing, target screening, in vitro diagnostics, and a wide range of applications in single-cell transcriptomics, proteomics, and metabolomics are emerging technologies, which are also faced with grand challenges and opportunities.

To help close the loop for research and development of precise treatment and early intervention, the integration of omics technology, bioinformatics, and AI technologies will facilitate technological innovation and clinical verification in the future of smart hospitals. We can foresee an increasing number of miniaturized, implantable, and intelligent medical robots in the near future.

1.5 Overview of This Book

These are some of the key elements that are covered in this book to provide a fresh and up-to-date overview of medical robotics. This book focuses on three areas of medical robotics: (1) robotic surgery (Chaps. 2 and 3), (2) rehabilitation robotics (Chaps. 4 and 5), and (3) hospital automation (Chap. 6). For each area, clinical needs and technical aspects will be discerned in detail, focusing on robotic systems and publications that represent key advances in medical robotics, thus providing the readers with an overview of the current state of the art. Open challenges and future directions are identified and discussed in Chap. 7. This book is intended to provide an overview of medical robotics by reporting on systems that have proceeded to clinical translation or commercialization from academia, highlighting their practical impact and innovation.

References

1. Driller J, Neumann G. An electromagnetic biopsy device. IEEE Trans Biomed Eng. 1967;1:52–3.
2. Bergeles C, Yang G-Z. From passive tool holders to microsurgeons: safer, smaller, smarter surgical robots. IEEE Trans Biomed Eng. 2013;61(5):1565–76.
3. Kwoh YS, Hou J, Jonckheere EA, et al. A robot with improved absolute positioning accuracy for CT guided stereotactic brain surgery. IEEE Trans Biomed Eng. 1988;35(2):153–60.
4. Troccaz J, Dagnino G, Yang G-Z. Frontiers of medical robotics: from concept to systems to clinical translation. Annu Rev Biomed Eng. 2019;21:193–218.
5. Vitiello V, Lee S-L, Cundy TP, et al. Emerging robotic platforms for minimally invasive surgery. IEEE Rev Biomed Eng. 2012;6:111–26.
6. Yang G-Z, Bergeles C, Vitiello V. Surgical robotics: the next 25 years: successes, challenges, and the road ahead. UK-RAS Network; 2016.
7. Payne CJ, Yang G-Z. Hand-held medical robots. Ann Biomed Eng. 2014;42(8):1594–605.
8. Cundy TP, Shetty K, Clark J, et al. The first decade of robotic surgery in children. J Pediatr Surg. 2013;48(4):858–65.
9. Marcus HJ, Cundy TP, Nandi D, et al. Robot-assisted and fluoroscopy-guided pedicle screw placement: a systematic review. Eur Spine J. 2014;23(2):291–7.

10. Lee S-L, Lerotic M, Vitiello V, et al. From medical images to minimally invasive intervention: computer assistance for robotic surgery. Comput Med Imaging Graph. 2010;34(1):33–45.
11. Marcus HJ, Hughes-Hallett A, Payne CJ, et al. Trends in the diffusion of robotic surgery: a retrospective observational study. Int J Med Robot Comput Assist Surg. 2017;13(4):e1870.
12. Karimyan V, Sodergren M, Clark J, et al. Navigation systems and platforms in natural orifice translumenal endoscopic surgery. Int J Surg. 2009;7(4):297–304.
13. Rafii-Tari H, Payne CJ, Yang G-Z. Current and emerging robot-assisted endovascular catheterization technologies: a review. Ann Biomed Eng. 2014;42(4):697–715.
14. Lavallee S, Troccaz J, Gaborit L, et al. Image guided operating robot: a clinical application in stereotactic neurosurgery. In: Proceedings of the IEEE international conference on robotics and automation, 1992. IEEE Computer Society; 1992.
15. Paul HA, Bargar WL, Mittlestadt B, et al. Development of a surgical robot for cementless total hip arthroplasty. Clin Orthop Relat Res. 1992;285:57–66.
16. Butner SE, Ghodoussi M. Transforming a surgical robot for human telesurgery. IEEE Trans Robot Autom. 2003;19(5):818–24.
17. Marescaux J, Leroy J, Gagner M, et al. Transatlantic robot-assisted telesurgery. Nature. 2001;413(6854):379–80.
18. Yaxley JW, Coughlin GD, Chambers SK, et al. Robot-assisted laparoscopic prostatectomy versus open radical retropubic prostatectomy: early outcomes from a randomised controlled phase 3 study. Lancet. 2016;388(10049):1057–66.
19. Di Biase L, Wang Y, Horton R, et al. Ablation of atrial fibrillation utilizing robotic catheter navigation in comparison to manual navigation and ablation: single-center experience. J Cardiovasc Electrophysiol. 2009;20(12):1328–35.
20. Riga CV, Bicknell CD, Rolls A, et al. Robot-assisted fenestrated endovascular aneurysm repair (FEVAR) using the Magellan system. J Vasc Interv Radiol. 2013;24(2):191–6.
21. Shang J, Noonan DP, Payne C, et al. An articulated universal joint based flexible access robot for minimally invasive surgery. In: Proceedings of the 2011 IEEE international conference on robotics and automation. IEEE; 2011.
22. Newton RC, Noonan DP, Vitiello V, et al. Robot-assisted transvaginal peritoneoscopy using confocal endomicroscopy: a feasibility study in a porcine model. Surg Endosc. 2012;26(9):2532–40.
23. Sears P, Dupont P. A steerable needle technology using curved concentric tubes. In: Proceedings of the 2006 IEEE/RSJ international conference on intelligent robots and systems. IEEE; 2006.
24. Webster RJ III. Design and mechanics of continuum robots for surgery. Baltimore, MD: Johns Hopkins University; 2008.
25. Furusho J, Ono T, Murai R, et al. Development of a curved multi-tube (CMT) catheter for percutaneous umbilical blood sampling and control methods of CMT catheters for solid organs. In: Proceedings of the IEEE International Conference Mechatronics and Automation, 2005. IEEE; 2005.
26. Dupont PE, Lock J, Itkowitz B, et al. Design and control of concentric-tube robots. IEEE Trans Robot. 2009;26(2):209–25.
27. Webster RJ, Swensen JP, Romano JM, et al. Closed-form differential kinematics for concentric-tube continuum robots with application to visual servoing. In: Khatib O, Kumar V, Pappas GJ, editors. Experimental robotics. Berlin: Springer; 2009. p. 485–94.
28. Arabagi V, Gosline A, Wood RJ, et al. Simultaneous soft sensing of tissue contact angle and force for millimeter-scale medical robots. In: Proceedings of the 2013 IEEE international conference on robotics and automation. IEEE; 2013.
29. Burgner J, Rucker DC, Gilbert HB, et al. A telerobotic system for transnasal surgery. IEEE/ASME Trans Mechatron. 2013;19(3):996–1006.
30. Valdastri P, Simi M, Webster RJ III. Advanced technologies for gastrointestinal endoscopy. Annu Rev Biomed Eng. 2012;14:397–429.
31. Gorini S, Quirini M, Menciassi A, et al. A novel SMA-based actuator for a legged endoscopic capsule. In: Proceedings of the The first IEEE/RAS-EMBS international conference on biomedical robotics and biomechatronics, 2006 BioRob 2006. IEEE; 2006.

32. Kwon J, Park S, Park J, et al. Evaluation of the critical stroke of an earthworm-like robot for capsule endoscopes. Proc Inst Mech Eng H J Eng Med. 2007;221(4):397–405.
33. Popek KM, Hermans T, Abbott JJ. First demonstration of simultaneous localization and propulsion of a magnetic capsule in a lumen using a single rotating magnet. In: Proceedings of the 2017 IEEE international conference on robotics and automation (ICRA). IEEE; 2017.
34. Iddan G, Meron G, Glukhovsky A, et al. Wireless capsule endoscopy. Nature. 2000;405(6785):417.
35. Beard JR, Officer A, De Carvalho IA, et al. The World report on ageing and health: a policy framework for healthy ageing. Lancet. 2016;387(10033):2145–54.
36. Gorelick PB. The global burden of stroke: persistent and disabling. Lancet Neurol. 2019;18(5):417–8.
37. Livingston G, Huntley J, Sommerlad A, et al. Dementia prevention, intervention, and care: 2020 report of the Lancet Commission. Lancet. 2020;396(10248):413–46.
38. Yang G-Z, Riener R, Dario P. To integrate and to empower: robots for rehabilitation and assistance. Am Assoc Adv Sci. 2017;2:eaan5593.
39. Matarić MJ. Socially assistive robotics: human augmentation versus automation. Sci Robot. 2017;2(4):eaam5410.
40. Broekens J, Heerink M, Rosendal H. Assistive social robots in elderly care: a review. Geron. 2009;8(2):94–103.
41. Mendez V, Iberite F, Shokur S, et al. Current solutions and future trends for robotic prosthetic hands. Ann Rev Control Robot Auton Syst. 2021;4:595–627.
42. Brose SW, Weber DJ, Salatin BA, et al. The role of assistive robotics in the lives of persons with disability. Am J Phys Med Rehabil. 2010;89(6):509–21.
43. Topping M. An overview of the development of handy 1, a rehabilitation robot to assist the severely disabled. J Intell Robot Syst. 2002;34:253–63.
44. Hidler J, Nichols D, Pelliccio M, et al. Advances in the understanding and treatment of stroke impairment using robotic devices. Top Stroke Rehabil. 2005;12(2):22–35.
45. Burgar CG, Lum PS, Shor PC, et al. Development of robots for rehabilitation therapy: the Palo Alto VA/Stanford experience. J Rehabil Res Dev. 2000;37(6):663–74.
46. Riener R, Lünenburger L, Colombo G. Human-centered robotics applied to gait training and assessment. J Rehabil Res Dev. 2006;43(5):679–94.
47. Keller U, Schölch S, Albisser U, et al. Robot-assisted arm assessments in spinal cord injured patients: a consideration of concept study. PLoS One. 2015;10(5):e0126948.
48. Krebs HI, Hogan N, Aisen ML, et al. Robot-aided neurorehabilitation. IEEE Trans Rehabil Eng. 1998;6(1):75–87.
49. Nef T, Mihelj M, Riener R. ARMin: a robot for patient-cooperative arm therapy. Med Biol Eng Comput. 2007;45(9):887–900.
50. Jezernik S, Colombo G, Keller T, et al. Robotic orthosis lokomat: a rehabilitation and research tool. Neuromodulation. 2003;6(2):108–15.
51. Guo Y, Gu X, Yang G-Z. Human–robot interaction for rehabilitation robotics. In: Glauner P, Plugmann P, Lerzynski G, editors. Digitalization in healthcare. Cham: Springer; 2021. p. 269–95.
52. Chaudhary U, Birbaumer N, Ramos-Murguialday A. Brain–computer interfaces for communication and rehabilitation. Nat Rev Neurol. 2016;12(9):513–25.
53. Esquenazi A, Talaty M, Packel A, et al. The ReWalk powered exoskeleton to restore ambulatory function to individuals with thoracic-level motor-complete spinal cord injury. Am J Phys Med Rehabil. 2012;91(11):911–21.
54. Angold HKR, Harding N, Richmond K, et al. Ekso bionics-Ekso bionics. IEEE Spectr. 2015;49(1):30–2.
55. Sankai Y. HAL: hybrid assistive limb based on cybernics. In: Kaneko M, Nakamura Y, editors. Robotics research. Berlin: Springer; 2010. p. 25–34.
56. Von Haxthausen F, Böttger S, Wulff D, et al. Medical robotics for ultrasound imaging: current systems and future trends. Curr Robot Rep. 2021;2(1):55–71.

57. Yang G-ZJ, Nelson B, Murphy RR, et al. Combating COVID-19—the role of robotics in managing public health and infectious diseases. Am Assoc Adv Sci. 2020;5:eabb5589.
58. Gao A, Murphy RR, Chen W, et al. Progress in robotics for combating infectious diseases. Sci Robot. 2021;6(52):eabf1462.
59. Kovach CR, Taneli Y, Neiman T, et al. Evaluation of an ultraviolet room disinfection protocol to decrease nursing home microbial burden, infection and hospitalization rates. BMC Infect Dis. 2017;17(1):1–8.
60. Eickmann M, Gravemann U, Handke W, et al. Inactivation of three emerging viruses–severe acute respiratory syndrome coronavirus, Crimean–Congo haemorrhagic fever virus and Nipah virus–in platelet concentrates by ultraviolet C light and in plasma by methylene blue plus visible light. Vox Sang. 2020;115(3):146–51.
61. Rodriguez-Gonzalez CG, Herranz-Alonso A, Escudero-Vilaplana V, et al. Robotic dispensing improves patient safety, inventory management, and staff satisfaction in an outpatient hospital pharmacy. J Eval Clin Pract. 2019;25(1):28–35.
62. Alahmari AR, Alrabghi KK, Dighriri IM. An overview of the current state and perspectives of pharmacy robot and medication dispensing technology. Cureus. 2022;14(8):e28642.
63. Tsukahara A, Kawanishi R, Hasegawa Y, et al. Sit-to-stand and stand-to-sit transfer support for complete paraplegic patients with robot suit HAL. Adv Robot. 2010;24(11):1615–38.
64. Jacob M, Li Y-T, Akingba G, et al. Gestonurse: a robotic surgical nurse for handling surgical instruments in the operating room. J Robot Surg. 2012;6(1):53–63.
65. Gu E, Tang X, Langner S, et al. Robot-based high-throughput screening of antisolvents for lead halide perovskites. Joule. 2020;4(8):1806–22.
66. Shental N, Levy S, Wuvshet V, et al. Efficient high-throughput SARS-CoV-2 testing to detect asymptomatic carriers. Sci Adv. 2020;6(37):eabc5961.
67. Twinanda AP, Shehata S, Mutter D, et al. Endonet: a deep architecture for recognition tasks on laparoscopic videos. IEEE Trans Med Imaging. 2016;36(1):86–97.
68. Yang G-Z, Cambias J, Cleary K, et al. Medical robotics—regulatory, ethical, and legal considerations for increasing levels of autonomy. Am Assoc Adv Sci. 2017;2:eaam8638.
69. Yang G-Z, Bellingham J, Dupont PE, et al. The grand challenges of science robotics. Sci Robot. 2018;3(14):eaar7650.
70. Berg J, Lu S. Review of interfaces for industrial human-robot interaction. Curr Robot Rep. 2020;1(2):27–34.
71. Edsinger A, Kemp CC. Human-robot interaction for cooperative manipulation: handing objects to one another. In: Proceedings of the RO-MAN 2007-The 16th IEEE international symposium on robot and human interactive communication. IEEE; 2007.
72. Huang B, Vandini A, Hu Y, et al. A vision-guided dual arm sewing system for stent graft manufacturing. In: Proceedings of the 2016 IEEE/RSJ international conference on intelligent robots and systems (IROS). IEEE; 2016.
73. Adamides G, Christou G, Katsanos C, et al. Usability guidelines for the design of robot teleoperation: a taxonomy. IEEE Trans Hum Mach Syst. 2014;45(2):256–62.
74. Breazeal C, Dautenhahn K, Kanda T. Social robotics. In: Siciliano B, Khatib O, editors. Springer handbook of robotics. Cham: Springer; 2016. p. 1935–72.
75. Adolphs R. Cognitive neuroscience of human social behaviour. Nat Rev Neurosci. 2003;4(3):165–78.
76. Jain S, Thiagarajan B, Shi Z, et al. Modeling engagement in long-term, in-home socially assistive robot interventions for children with autism spectrum disorders. Sci Robot. 2020;5(39):eaaz3791.
77. Scassellati B, Boccanfuso L, Huang C-M, et al. Improving social skills in children with ASD using a long-term, in-home social robot. Sci Robot. 2018;3(21):eaat7544.
78. Yang G-Z, Dario P, Kragic D. Social robotics—trust, learning, and social interaction. Am Assoc Adv Sci. 2018;3:eaau8839.

Robotic Surgery 2

Contents

2.1 Introduction

This chapter presents an overview of the clinical aspects that influence the design, development, and uptake of surgical robots. It mainly focuses on the evolution of surgery and related clinical technologies, reporting clinical applications of robotic surgery, and analyzing clinical needs and challenges that are relevant to the translation and usability of robotic technologies in clinical practice. The goal is to provide readers with an overall view of clinical requirements that are needed to design robotic systems for surgical applications. Technical aspects of robotic surgery, including the state of the art of surgical robotic platforms and analysis of general technologies (i.e., imaging, sensing, navigation, control, human–robot interaction, and autonomy), will be covered in Chap. 3.

The field of surgery is under constant evolution [1] (see Fig. 2.1) with an accelerated pace in recent years in terms of safety, effectiveness, and patient outcome. This process started a long time ago with the introduction of antiseptic surgery by Lister in the 1860s. Since then, the discovery of breakthrough technologies has played an important role in revolutionizing clinical practices such as surgery, anesthesiology, radiology, and many others. While technical advancements clearly improve the

Y. Guo et al., *Medical Robotics*, Innovative Medical Devices,
https://doi.org/10.1007/978-981-99-7317-0_2

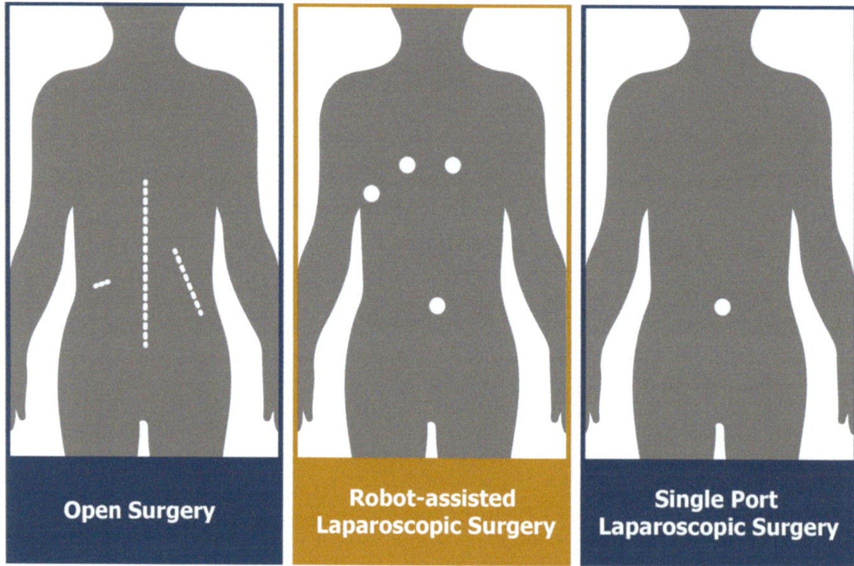

Fig. 2.1 The evolution of surgery is strictly linked to the evolution of technology. Advanced medical imaging coupled with smaller, flexible, and more dexterous instruments and sensing devices allowed the move from open to minimally invasive approaches, reducing the number and size of surgical wounds, thus soft tissue damages, surgical infection incidence, recovery time, and postoperative pain

strategies for the diagnosis and treatment of a growing number of pathologies, the core of surgical practice remains basically unchanged and focuses on high-level performances and technical rigor. Driven by technological breakthroughs, this founding surgical principle has undergone a dramatic and quick evolution in the last decades, and new exciting developments are predicted in coming years.

The era of MIS was initiated by the development of the Hopkins' endoscope in the 60s. Then, MIS underwent a formative period of clinical assessment and technological progression in the 1970s and 1980s before becoming established across several surgical specialties. MIS continues to focus on minimizing the number and size of visible skin incisions, with the goal of thus improving the surgical outcome (e.g., reducing postoperative pain, surgical and recovery time, risk of infections, etc.).

While MIS has a clear benefit to patients, it requires surgeons to acquire new skills to operate novel tools in different surgical workflows with respect to standard open surgery. The main changes are related to sight and touch, possibly the two most important senses for surgeons. During MIS, the 2D video display of the surgical field and the rigid laparoscopes represents a barrier between the surgeon and the patient as haptic guidance, hand dexterity, and visual-motor coordination are drastically reduced. To mitigate such limitations, robotic surgical platforms have been introduced into clinical practice, bringing solutions such as enhanced dexterity and manipulability and improved stability and motion accuracy.

Robotic technologies combined with MIS approaches, allowed further reduction of skin incisions up to a single incision, or even no-incisions, by navigating the natural orifices of the human body to reach the target anatomies (see Fig. 2.1). One of the main goals is the possibility to navigate the human body in a flexible way, i.e., to reach anatomies that are not directly aligned to the access site. New technologies are required to make the "flexible access surgery" possible, and bespoke instrumentation with higher flexibility and dexterity to reach such anatomical target is therefore required.

2.2 Surgical Robots and Clinical Needs

Surgical robots were originally developed to address the clinical demand for greater accuracy in manipulation and visualization, overcoming the challenges of conventional minimally invasive approaches (ergonomically difficult to perform due to the use of rigid instruments, limited sensory feedback, misalignment of visuomotor axes, and the need for high dexterity). In response to these limitations, robotics and computer assistance have been integrated into the clinical workflow to provide augmentation of surgical skills in terms of enhanced dexterity, sensing, and image guidance [1].

As shown in Fig. 2.2, robotic systems have already been used in many specialties, including neurosurgery, ENT, orthopedics, laparoscopy and via human body lumens. According to Bergeles et al. [2], there are four generations of surgical robots: (1) stereotaxic robotic systems (first generation); (2) rigid dexterous robots for MIS (second generation); (3) flexible robots for MIS (third generation); and (4) untethered microsurgeons (fourth generation). Standard laparoscopy (manual) can be considered as the zeroth generation. From one generation to the next, the fusion of robotics and imaging became stronger and more effective, providing better support to the surgeons in terms of improved manipulation skill and precision as well as more effective surgical planning and intra-operative guidance.

2.2.1 Standard Laparoscopy

In laparoscopy, surgical tools are inserted and manipulated inside the abdomen through a number of small incisions. To facilitate the visualization of the surgical field and the manipulation of the instruments, the abdomen is inflated with CO_2. The first laparoscopic surgery in 1985, the removal of the gall bladder by Mühe in 1985 [4], marked the transition from open to minimally invasive surgery. Despite the aforementioned advantages, MIS faces significant application challenges, particularly in the newer surgical domains of single-port access, intraluminal, and transluminal surgery [1].

These complications revolve around ergonomic factors associated with limited sensory feedback of surgeons, i.e., misalignment of visuomotor axes and a high demand for manual dexterity required to manipulate the laparoscopic instruments.

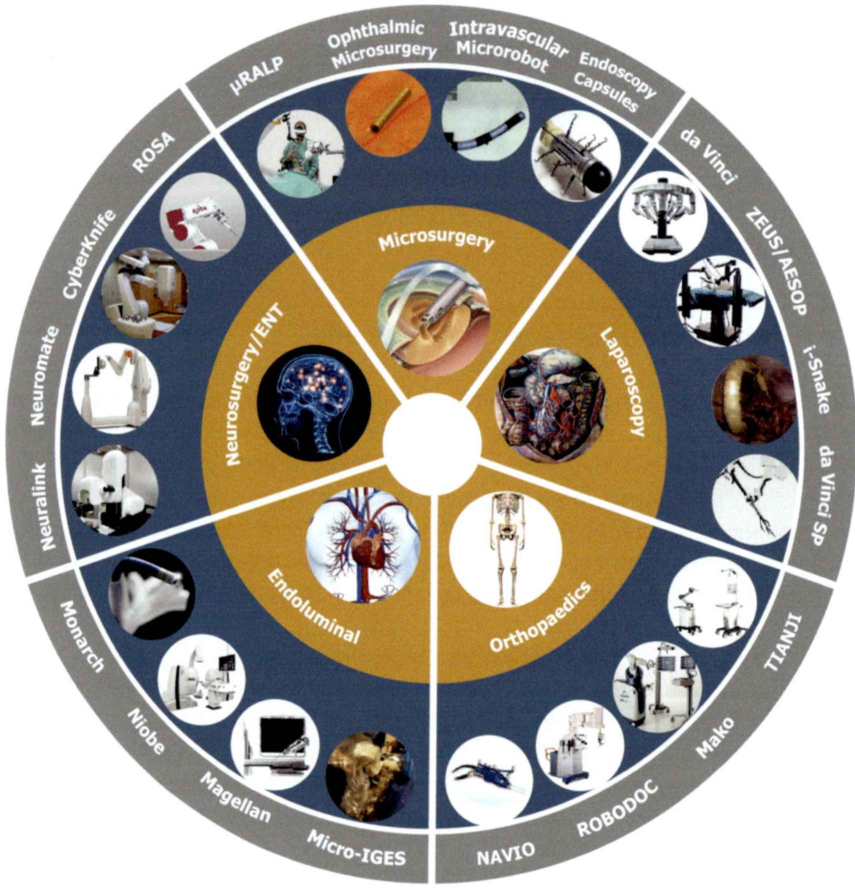

Fig. 2.2 Examples of surgical robot specializations. µRALP surgical system, Mattos et al. (µRALP Consortium; https://www.microralp.edu); Ophthalmic microsurgery/intravascular microrobot/endoscopy capsules (adapted with IEEE permission from [2]); da Vinci and da Vinci SP, Intuitive Surgical Inc., © 2023; ZEUS/AESOP, © Computer Motion; i-Snake (adapted with IEEE permission from [2]); NAVIO, Smith&Nephew, © 2023; ROBODOC, Creative Commons (CC BY 4.0); Mako, Stryker, © 2023; TIANJI, Beijing TINAVI Medical Technologies Co., Ltd., © 2020; Micro-IGES (adapted with IEEE permission from [3]); Monarch, Johnson&Johnson MedTech, © 2023; neuromate, Renishaw, © 2023; CyberKnife, Wikimedia Commons (CC BY 2.0); Neuralink, Neuralink, © 2023; ROSA ONE, Zimmer Biomet, © 2023

In more detail, in laparoscopy procedures, surgeons operate while looking at a screen displaying 2D images provided by the endoscope. Therefore, stereoscopic depth perception is commonly lost, and visual estimation skills are limited [5]. Haptic feedback is also limited as surgeons have to manipulate the surgical tools while tackling the fulcrum effect resulting from the constraining incision ports [6]. The lack of feedback makes certain types of surgeries particularly challenging. Endovascular intervention, for example, requires force feedback to navigate the human vasculature, rendering safe tissue manipulation highly demanding [7].

2.2.2 Neurosurgery and Orthopedics

The first generation of surgical robots was applied to stereotaxic neurosurgery and orthopedics. Rigid structures such as bones simplify the registration of preoperative images (e.g., CT or MRI) of the patient to the robotic platform, allowing for preoperative planning and intra-operative navigation in real-time. Exemplary systems for neurosurgery (which will be analyzed in more detail in the next chapter along with other surgical robot specializations) include the industrial robotic manipulator Puma 200 (Unimation, Danbury, USA) that was used in neurosurgical tasks as robot-assisted needle placement for brain biopsy. This is the first example in the history of a robot used for surgical applications [8]. Since then, surgical robots gradually steered away from industrial manipulators toward dedicated bespoke systems designed and developed for clinical applications. The *Neuromate* (available from Renishaw, New Mills, UK) [9] was the first surgical robot for neurosurgery that received *Conformité Européene* (CE) and FDA approval. "Minerva" is another example of a robot designed for neurosurgical applications [10].

Orthopedic surgical robots evolved in parallel to neurosurgical systems. ROBODOC, the first commercially successful surgical robot [11, 12], was developed by Taylor and Kazanzides et al. in IBM and commercialized by Integrated Surgical Systems Inc. ROBODOC, clinically evaluated in 1992, performed total hip replacement. In the UK, Davies and colleagues developed "AcroBot," a surgical robot for knee arthroplasty that was able to cooperate with surgeons providing active constraints [13].

This first generation of surgical robots allowed interventions of increased accuracy, and their success supported the acceptance of robots operating in surgical suites [2], representing the foundation of state-of-the-art robotic surgical systems [14]. Through iterations and building on existing research contributions, systems gradually became more lightweight and compact. They are, however, not designed to allow visualization, haptic feedback, or surgical dexterity in multiple DoF. These issues are key requirements for improving the outcome of minimally invasive interventions that involve tissue manipulation. This is the focus of the next generation of robotic systems, which are based on the integration of imaging modalities, the notion of synergistically operating with the surgeon, and the now-established limitations of surgical and robotic capabilities [2].

2.2.3 Robotic Laparoscopy and Endoluminal Intervention

Next generations of surgical robots approach the problem of operating in confined body cavities and dexterously manipulating tissue. The design of any MIS platform should therefore be aimed at simplifying the procedure for the surgeon. As suggested by Vitiello et al. [1], requirements for such platforms include accessing the endoluminal site; tissue manipulation and removal (e.g., resection or ablation); and tissue suturing.

Such platforms also require a small footprint to provide enhanced dexterity, precision, and stability and adequate visualization of the surgical workspace. Accordingly, minimally invasive access can be divided into the following categories [1]: extraluminal, intraluminal, and transluminal as summarized in Fig. 2.3. In extraluminal approaches, the access to the surgical field is obtained through skin incisions (one or more); endoluminal approaches utilize anatomical lumens via natural orifices, and transluminal procedures are performed by breaching luminal barrier to access the target anatomy. A combination of these three approaches is also possible (hybrid). Each approach presents a specific surgical configuration, generating a set of ergonomic and technical challenges.

Laparoscopy and thoracoscopy are examples of minimally invasive techniques that utilize extraluminal access routes to insert instruments via small incisions in the abdominal or chest wall (see Fig. 2.1). CO_2 gas is insufflated in the anatomical spaces to create the required operational space (particularly important for laparoscopy). Ergonomic challenges include counterintuitive tool manipulation due to the fulcrum effect and loss of dexterity due to the use of rigid instruments with limited effective workspace.

Single-port laparoscopy procedures have the benefit of reducing the number of skin incisions required for instrument access. Such procedures are usually carried out through an incision on the umbilicus through which laparoscopic instruments are inserted into the body. The main limitation of this approach is the instruments clashing due to the limited and "crowded" access that can be addressed by utilizing

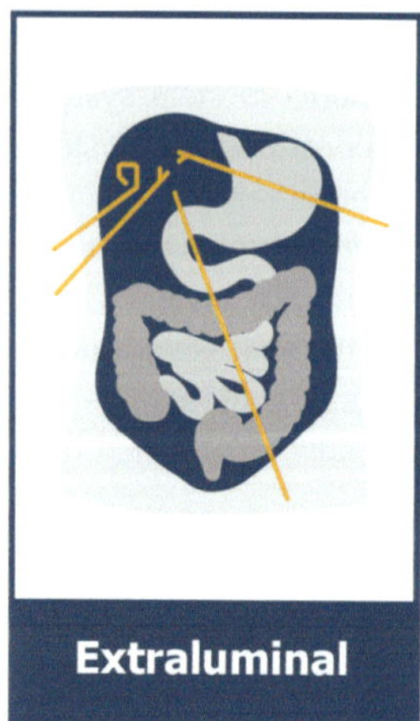

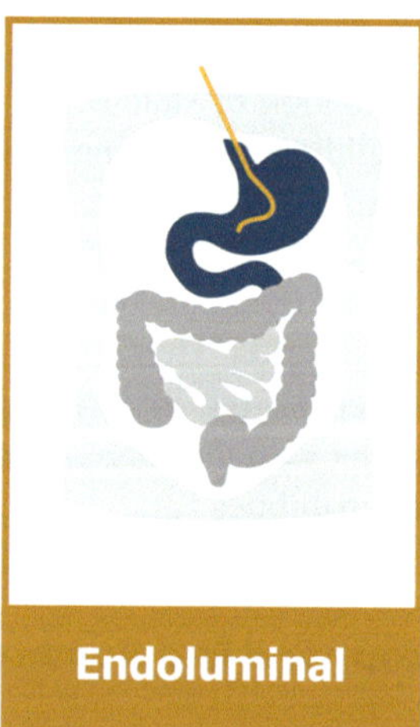

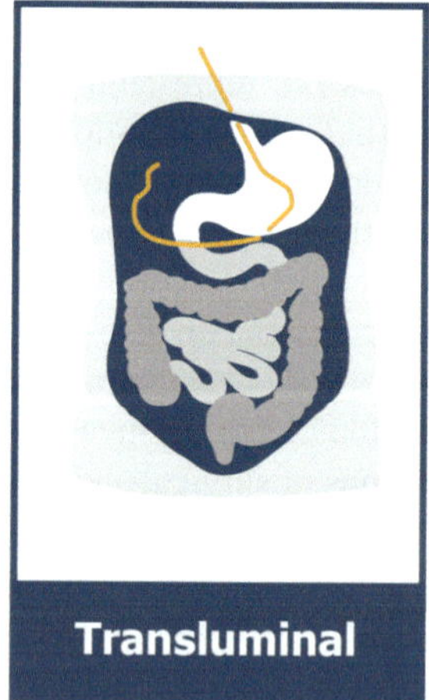

Fig. 2.3 Classification of MIS procedures. Based on the access routes, MIS procedures include extraluminal, intraluminal, and transluminal approaches. In extraluminal approaches, the instruments are inserted through skin incisions on the body. Endoluminal intervention makes use of the natural orifices of the human body to access lumens and navigate the instrument to the desired target. Transluminal access is provided by breaching a luminal barrier to enter into body cavities such as the abdomen. Hybrid approaches use a combination of these access routes

pre-curved instruments. However, the problem related to the rigidity of the shaft of such instruments remains.

Endoluminal procedures are performed through human lumens as the vascular tree, esophagus, urethra, and colon, without passing through their boundaries. Endoluminal devices, such as endoscopes and catheters, are used to navigate the lumens and deploy a therapy or perform a diagnosis. For example, in colonoscopy, an endoscope navigates the colon to provide images of the tissues and take out tissues (biopsy, polyp resection) [15]. In contrast to extraluminal procedures, intraluminal procedures are spatially constrained by the very limited operative workspace. Therefore, instrument flexibility is crucial for safe access and navigation.

Endovascular procedures are performed through blood vessels. 2D fluoroscopy is typically used as image guidance to navigate catheters and wires, and this introduces a number of challenges, such as exposure to x-ray radiations and suboptimal visualization of soft tissues, which requires the injection of a nephrotoxic contrast agent. Vascular instruments are manipulated by the operator (generally endovascular surgeons and interventional radiologists) to navigate arteries and reach a specific target to, for example, place a stent and perform aneurysm coiling, ablation, or drug delivery. Such procedures require the operator to be extremely skilled, and extensive training is required to reach the necessary level of manual dexterity. Thus, these drive the need for the development of robotic systems for endovascular intervention [16].

Transluminal approaches make use of flexible endoscopes to improve gastrointestinal and hepatobiliary surgeries, further minimizing the invasiveness of related MIS procedures. Endoscopes are inserted through a natural orifice and involve a breach of luminal barriers to reach the desired target, for example, the abdominal cavity. These approaches are called natural orifice transluminal endoscopic surgery (NOTES) and can involve a combination of transrectal transgastric, transvesical, or transvaginal routes requiring specific endoscopic instrumentation. However, the standard endoscopic instrumentation is not adequate for transluminal procedures. Attempted NOTES applications outside of normally supportive luminal boundaries reveal a lack of structural shape strength due to a tendency for the tip to wander away from the desired target. In addition, current surgical tools and devices compatible with flexible endoscopes cannot guarantee the required interaction capabilities with the tissue. Therefore, the design of tailored instruments is crucial to the clinical uptake of NOTES. Major technical challenges are related to the flexibility of instruments to allow navigation to the surgical site through different access routes while maintaining adequate stability. The goal is to meet the same capabilities of complex multihanded laparoscopic instruments to reproduce the abilities of human hands to perform open surgery. The integration of elements such as elevated optics coupled with independently controlled bimanual arms into such a platform design represents a major technical challenge.

A combination of extraluminal, endoluminal, and transluminal approaches—called hybrid approach—is possible. For example, a laparoscopic instrument can be deployed extraluminally to support procedures that involve transluminal access. Another example is related to cardiac surgery [17], where some tasks are via endovascular approach (e.g., stenting) in conjunction with extraluminal intervention, allowing a minimally invasive approach that otherwise would require open heart surgery and related invasive procedures (e.g., thoracotomy or sternotomy).

2.3 New Challenges, New Technologies

2.3.1 Superhuman Dexterity and Human–Robot Cooperation

In robotic surgery, many problems associated with conventional MIS are addressed by combining machine precision and human control. By using a digital, as opposed to mechanical, teleoperated setup—in which the clinical operators work with the main robot and the remote manipulator works with the patient— the fulcrum effect is eliminated. Tremor removal and motion scaling are used to control the instrument end-effector's motion precisely. Additional flexibility at the remote manipulator level enables wrist articulation.

The development of surgical robots takes into account not only their size and architecture but also their capacity to collaborate with the surgical team and safety features—crucial for clinical acceptance and usability. For safety and the best surgical outcome, it is essential to design an appropriate human–robot interface and specific control strategies. Medical robots were initially employed as passive tool holders (e.g., Neuronavigator [18]), but subsequently they became able to adjust preprogrammed plans in real-time to the intraoperative position of a target (e.g., CyberKnife [19]). The choice of a suitable human–robot interface and the application of task-specific control strategies are fundamental to the improvement of the consistency and safety of the operation, especially when the complexity of multi-DoF systems introduces additional ergonomic issues for the surgeon [1]. Although most of the current platforms are controlled in a teleoperated fashion, different human–robot interfaces and control features have also been implemented depending on specific designs and clinical applications. However, these components mainly affect the configuration of the operator side of the system unless additional constraints need to be introduced at the patient level.

2.3.2 Vision and Sensing in Robotic Surgery

To give operators superhuman dexterity and integrated real-time intraoperative image guidance, sensing, and decision support, surgical robotic platforms must seamlessly collaborate with surgeons. The surgeon closes the system's control loop and operates the robot by using sight and sense data. As a result, real-time imaging and sensing could be integrated in the control architecture to further improve the conventional teleoperated configuration (in which the remote robot within the patient replicates the movements of the surgeon's hands at the master controller) [14].

Video display (2D or 3D) that gives the surgeon visual feedback from the surgical site and an input device that transmits motion commands to the remote robot are the two essential parts of a surgical master console. The clinical process and the remote manipulator's design are key factors that influence the input device selection. Joysticks and the PHANTOM Omni haptic devices are common examples of off-the-shelf components used in simple surgical systems. A bespoke control mechanism is typically necessary for systems with several degrees of freedom. However, redundancy makes it difficult to develop an ergonomic user interface since human hands can only handle three degrees of freedom at once, necessitating the independent control of extra degrees of freedom. Perceptual docking, a method introduced by Yang et al. [20], can be used to enhance the surgeon's control of the robot. This conceptualization makes use of sensing to learn from the visuo-motor activity of the users. This paradigm makes use of binocular eye-tracking to gather in-depth data about the subject's eye gaze. Exemplary applications include recovering 3D motion and soft tissue deformation using this information [21]. As a result, this methodology can be integrated into the robotic control to provide visual stabilization and motion correction [22]. In order to lessen the cognitive load on the surgeon and increase procedural safety, perceptual docking leverages the eye gaze to generate active haptic constraints [23].

As already indicated, a primary flaw with many surgical devices continues to be the absence of haptic guidance and force control. A robotic master control device may render haptic feedback to give surgeons the perceptual information needed for navigation and effective force delivery. The surgeon can use instrument-induced tissue deformation as visual feedback to infer the amount of force used. When executing technically more difficult and delicate surgical activities, such as manipulating sutures, haptic feedback becomes increasingly important [24].

Okamura and colleagues conducted in-depth research to demonstrate the critical function of haptic feedback in robotic surgery [25]. In addition to a number of force and position-based impedance control strategies for teleoperation [26] and the development of virtual fixtures [27] (more on this below), they have looked into the use of visuo-auditory cues [28, 29], to balance the lack of haptic guidance. However, sensory substitution is less effective than direct haptic guidance because operators have to "translate" the visuo-auditory information into a force estimation. Additionally, it is still a significant challenge to use sensory substitution to transmit information from a large number of DoFs [30].

Virtual fixtures (or active constraints) can also improve the surgeon's sensory feedback by directing the surgical tool along predetermined 3D trajectories [31] and inside secure boundaries [32]. The Acrobot is one example of a robotic system that makes use of virtual fixtures [13]. Acrobot has a force feedback handle that is situated close to its end-effector. Through the handle, the surgeon may distinguish between cutting hard or soft tissue. The method does not need any force sensors and instead uses CT data acquired preoperatively. The surgeon can pre-plan the procedure using such imaging data and establish a safety region in which it is safe to remove bone tissue. When the end-effector approaches such region, the active constraint control increases the haptic stiffness to the surgeon's hand via the handle.

Active constraints' primary drawback is that they strongly rely on preoperative imaging data [32] and the accuracy of its intraoperative registration [33]. Dynamic virtual fixtures have been suggested to deal with dynamic surgical scenarios. For instance, Ren and colleagues created a 3D dynamic map of the surgical scenario by integrating CT and MRI data with intra-operative ultrasound [34]. However, the efficacy of such procedures still depends on the accurate registration of the preoperative model to the patient, which is usually limited by tissue deformations due to manipulation during surgery.

Instead of restricting merely the instrument tip, dynamic active constraints can be applied to give manipulation bounds to the entire robot [35], providing increased instrument control and safety, particularly when the constrained surgical workspace increases the complexity of the manipulation (e.g., in endoluminal procedures) [36].

More recently, Dagnino et al. proposed the concept of vision-based haptic feedback in endovascular procedures [7, 37, 38]. The robotic platform developed at Imperial College London, the CathBot system, allows for the robotic manipulation of endovascular instruments (catheters and guidewires), providing real-time intraoperative navigation, including visual and haptic guidance. In order to constrain the mobility of the endovascular instruments and direct the operator through the vascular tree, the navigation system analyzes the video stream provided by the imaging device (such as a fluoroscope or an MRI) and generates dynamic active constraints. This friction-like haptic guidance—generated through a robotic master manipulator—is calculated by continuously monitoring the relative positions of the instrument and the vessel walls. The friction felt by the user in the master manipulator increases as the instrument gets closer to the vessel wall. This avoids peak-force contacts between the instruments and the vessel walls, thus reducing the risk of injuries.

2.3.3 Image-Guided Robotic Surgery

The huge impact that medical imaging (together with surgical instrumentations) had on the field of surgery should now be clear to the reader. It constitutes a real breakthrough toward safer, more consistent, and minimally invasive intervention. The use of preoperative and intraoperative imaging augmented by robot-assisted instruments (see Fig. 2.4) has significantly improved surgeons' perceptual-motor capabilities, allowing surgical procedures to be carried out with unprecedented accuracy and efficiency [33].

Medical images are usually assessed preoperatively to plan the surgery. Intraoperative real-time imaging is important to guide the surgeon during the execution of the surgery. However, precise registration of the patient's anatomy with the preoperative data is necessary to enable real-time visual guidance. Registration can be carried out preoperatively and maintained constant throughout the surgery if deformations or changes in the tissues do not occur (like in fracture surgery). It is required to enable online registration and remodeling of the data if there is significant tissue deformation during the operation. For instance, due to its intricate structure and mobility, heart surgery continues to be challenging in this regard.

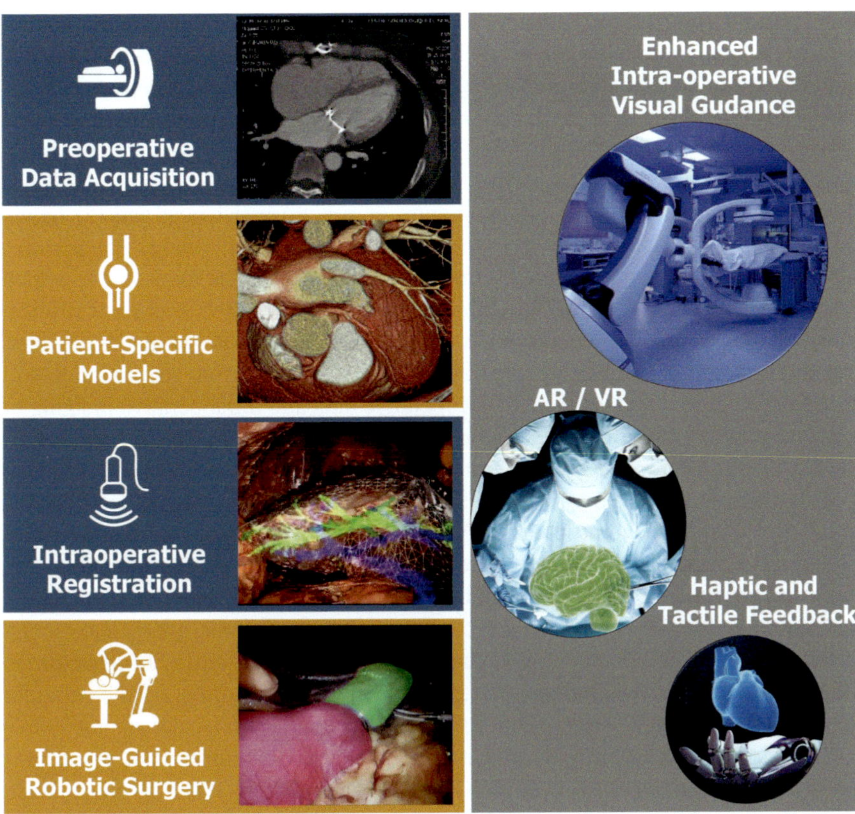

Fig. 2.4 Image-guided robotic surgery. Merging preoperative and intraoperative images augmented by robotic devices improves surgeons' perceptual-motor capabilities, allowing surgical procedures to be carried out with unprecedented accuracy and efficiency. Typical steps include the preoperative acquisition of patient's volumetric data (usually via MRI and/or CT) that are used to create patient-specific atlas and plan the procedure. Such a plan is then adapted in real-time during the surgical procedure according to intraoperative data (provided, for example, by ultrasound or fluoroscopy imaging). Co-registration of preoperative and intraoperative data, together with dynamic information such as tissue deformation and topological change, enables the implementation of robotic assistance for enhanced dexterity and motion control, as well as other important features such as enhanced surgical guidance via real-time 3D imaging, augmented and virtual reality, and haptic and tactile sensing with dynamic active constraints to improve the consistency and safety of the surgical procedures

Preoperative data collection is generally the initial stage in an image-guided surgical navigation system. A kinematic model of the robot, geometrical information for co-registration of preoperative planning, and simulation of alternative intraoperative approaches are three sources of information that must be combined in the case of robot-assisted MIS. The preoperative surgical plan is then modified in accordance with intraoperative information. Dynamic data, such as tissue deformation and topological change, is crucial in this regard. These data can be used to co-register preoperative and intraoperative data and make it easier to use *Augmented*

Reality (AR), for example, to map imaging data to the surgical field. Haptic boundaries are set and modified at this point if virtual fixtures are to be included. Procedure simulation can be used to evaluate the potential impact of surgical steps prior to its execution, albeit it is not yet common. In order to achieve its overall objectives, image-guided surgery must provide (1) pre-planning of the procedure; (2) intraoperative guidance through real-time imaging; (3) real-time tracking of the tissue deformation and adaptation; (4) integration of robotic assistance; and (5) haptic guidance and dynamic active constraints. For example, by combining intraoperative imaging and patient-specific models into a robotic platform, the robot can be guided through a pre-planned path [39]. Clinical requirements for robot-assisted surgical navigation include identification and localization of the pathology, spatial positioning and orientation (tissue and surgical tools), depth perception, adaptation to soft tissue deformation, and merging of preoperative data and intraoperative imaging or video stream [1]. Intraoperative tracking of tissues that deform can be made possible with the use of image guidance. Surgical workflow uses intraoperative imaging to provide tissue surfaces to the clinician, most frequently via endoscopy, fluoroscopy, or ultrasound. In particular, vision and guidance can be aided by the use of preoperative models and intraoperative imaging. Contrary to preoperative imaging, however, intraoperative real-time data collection is limited. Ultrasound imaging is affordable and widely available and can be used for soft tissue identification and guidance in MIS. Fluoroscopy is commonly used for orthopedics but is unable to show soft tissues unless iodine contrast is injected, for example, in endovascular applications (without the use of contrast, vessel, and other soft tissues are not visible to the operator). Real-time MRI guidance has been used to guide cardiac procedures [16], where *Magnetic Resonance* (MR) is able to provide good soft tissue contrast. While MRI is able to depict versatile tissue contrast, it is only possible to obtain a limited number of 2D images to attain the required temporal resolution. Also, MR-safe devices (e.g., the CathBot system for endovascular intervention) are required for any intervention within an MR scanner [38]. The development of MR-compatible robots is expected to be an exciting step forward in the field.

As mentioned above, the combination of both preoperative models and the intraoperative data and scene is necessary for effective intraoperative navigation. Registration to the intraoperative workspace is necessary for preoperative models to enable intraoperative guidance. Since the patients often require various imaging modalities, image registration and fusion between such modalities are also very important [40].

A prerequisite of image registration and visual navigation in robot-assisted surgical procedures is to accurately track the tissues (and their deformations, in the case of soft tissues) so that closed-loop control can be applied (e.g., vison-based control or visual servoing). Tracking of tissues involves two types of landmarks: (1) artificial landmarks (often referred to as fiducials) are external fiducials with definite shape, and (2) natural landmarks are tissue-specific local features on the tissue surface. These landmarks offer a reliable frame of reference that allows for image registration. However, tracking soft tissues during surgery is still difficult [33] mostly due to their free-form deformation and visually disparate surgical sceneries.

Natural landmarks deform with the surrounding structure, and the tracking consistency is generally sub-optimal. Assessing the relationship of the robot to the surrounding anatomy is also essential. In particular, the interaction of the entire robot with surrounding anatomical structures must be considered for safety reasons, i.e., to prevent injuries to the patient.

Finally, another important aspect is the augmentation of the surgical scene by including preoperatively and intraoperatively images and 3D models. In standard practice, preoperative information is examined before a procedure and then shown on a screen during the surgery. Now, preoperative or intraoperative data can be superimposed over the exposed surgical view using augmented reality. This is possible during orthopedics and neurosurgical applications where rigid structures like bones allow solid and consistent image registration, enabling the augmentation of the surgical field. However, this is still difficult in procedures where the deformation of soft tissue is important due to the limited registration of pre- and intra-operative data to the patient [1, 33].

2.4 Conclusions

Surgery is quickly evolving, driven by rapid technological advances and our continual search for early intervention and least invasive treatments. This chapter has provided an overview of the evolution of surgery and related clinical technologies, focusing on clinical needs and challenges that are relevant to the development and clinical uptake of surgical robotic platforms. Clinical challenges of minimally invasive surgeries are mainly related to surgical instruments that are ergonomically difficult due to the use of rigid instruments, surgical navigation (i.e., the limited sensory feedback and the misalignment of visuomotor axes), and the need for high dexterity.

For neurosurgery and orthopedics, it is crucial to provide reliable and consistent intraoperative navigation, where 3D preoperative images of the patient (e.g., CT and/or MRI) are registered to the patient to guide the clinical team during the surgery. Also, high precision (e.g., to place a needle in the brain or to mill a bone to place a prosthesis) and force (e.g., to reduce a joint fracture) are key aspects.

For laparoscopy, the main clinical challenge is operating in confined body cavities and dexterously manipulating tissue. Here, clinical requirements include the need for high dexterity, precision, stability, and an adequate visualization of the surgical workspace. For endoluminal procedures (i.e., performed through tubular anatomical structures such as the esophagus, colon, urethra, and arteries), the challenge is even more complex, as the instrument must be able to navigate an even smaller anatomical workspace and therefore instrument flexibility and steerability are crucial for safe access and navigation. On top of that, image and haptic guidance play a fundamental role in surgical navigation. For example, in endovascular procedures (which are examples of endoluminal intervention), 2D fluoroscopy is typically used as image guidance to navigate catheters and wires, but this introduces a number of challenges. 2D representation of a 3D anatomy is suboptimal, and it requires a nephrotoxic contrast agent to visualize soft tissues. X-ray radiations are not healthy for both the patient and the operator. Also, the operators rely on haptic feedback perceived through the instruments in order to navigate the instrument through the anatomy. Finally, the necessary proficiency in manual dexterity requires a wealth of training and experience.

New advances in the field of robotics, imaging, sensing, and AI can provide the necessary technologies and instruments to address the discussed clinical challenges. Building on the clinical considerations presented in this chapter, the next chapter will provide a detailed explanation of robotic surgery, outlining the evolution of robotic platforms and related technologies that have contributed to making robotic surgery a major area of innovation and development in the last decades.

References

1. Vitiello V, Lee S-L, Cundy TP, et al. Emerging robotic platforms for minimally invasive surgery. IEEE Rev Biomed Eng. 2012;6:111–26.
2. Bergeles C, Yang G-Z. From passive tool holders to microsurgeons: safer, smaller, smarter surgical robots. IEEE Trans Biomed Eng. 2013;61(5):1565–76.
3. Shang J, Leibrandt K, Giataganas P, et al. A single-port robotic system for transanal microsurgery—design and validation. IEEE Robot Automat Lett. 2017;2(3):1510–7.
4. Reynolds JRW. The first laparoscopic cholecystectomy. JSLS. 2001;5(1):89.
5. Tanagho YS, Andriole GL, Paradis AG, et al. 2D versus 3D visualization: impact on laparoscopic proficiency using the fundamentals of laparoscopic surgery skill set. J Laparoendosc Adv Surg Tech A. 2012;22(9):865–70.
6. Gallagher A, McClure N, McGuigan J, et al. An ergonomic analysis of the fulcrum effect in the acquisition of endoscopic skills. Endoscopy. 1998;30(07):617–20.
7. Dagnino G, Liu J, Abdelaziz ME, et al. Haptic feedback and dynamic active constraints for robot-assisted endovascular catheterization. In: Proceedings of the 2018 IEEE/RSJ international conference on intelligent robots and systems (IROS). IEEE; 2018.
8. Kwoh YS, Hou J, Jonckheere EA, et al. A robot with improved absolute positioning accuracy for CT guided stereotactic brain surgery. IEEE Trans Biomed Eng. 1988;35(2):153–60.
9. Lavallee S, Troccaz J, Gaborit L, et al. Image guided operating robot: a clinical application in stereotactic neurosurgery. In: Proceedings of the 1992 IEEE international conference on robotics and automation. IEEE Computer Society; 1992.
10. Glauser D, Fankhauser H, Epitaux M, et al. Neurosurgical robot Minerva: first results and current developments. J Image Guid Surg. 1995;1(5):266–72.
11. Paul HA, Mittlestadt B, Bargar WL, et al. A surgical robot for total hip replacement surgery. In: Proceedings of the ICRA. 1992.
12. Taylor RH, Mittelstadt BD, Paul HA, et al. An image-directed robotic system for precise orthopaedic surgery. IEEE Trans Robot Autom. 1994;10(3):261–75.
13. Jakopec MY, Baena FR, Harris SJ, et al. The hands-on orthopaedic robot "Acrobot": early clinical trials of total knee replacement surgery. IEEE Trans Robot Autom. 2003;19(5):902–11.
14. Troccaz J, Dagnino G, Yang G-Z. Frontiers of medical robotics: from concept to systems to clinical translation. Annu Rev Biomed Eng. 2019;21:193–218.
15. Ponsky J. Endoluminal surgery: past, present and future. Surg Endosc Other Interv Tech. 2006;20(2):S500–S2.
16. Rafii-Tari H, Payne CJ, Yang G-Z. Current and emerging robot-assisted endovascular catheterization technologies: a review. Ann Biomed Eng. 2014;42(4):697–715.
17. Hjortdal VE, Redington A, de Leval M, et al. Hybrid approaches to complex congenital cardiac surgery. Eur J Cardiothorac Surg. 2002;22(6):885–90.
18. Kosugi Y, Watanabe E, Goto J, et al. An articulated neurosurgical navigation system using MRI and CT images. IEEE Trans Biomed Eng. 1988;35(2):147–52.

19. Schweikard A, Shiomi H, Adler J. Respiration tracking in radiosurgery without fiducials. Int J Med Robot Comput Assist Surg. 2005;1(2):19–27.
20. Yang G-Z, Mylonas GP, Kwok K-W, et al. Perceptual docking for robotic control. In: Dohi T, Sakuma I, Liao H, editors. Medical imaging and virtual reality. Berlin: Springer; 2008. p. 21–30.
21. Mylonas GP, Stoyanov D, Deligianni F, et al. Gaze-contingent soft tissue deformation tracking for minimally invasive robotic surgery. In: Duncan JS, Gerig G, editors. Medical image computing and computer-assisted intervention. Berlin: Springer; 2005. p. 843–50.
22. Mylonas GP, Darzi A, Zhong Yang G. Gaze-contingent control for minimally invasive robotic surgery. Comput Aided Surg. 2006;11(5):256–66.
23. Mylonas GP, Kwok K-W, James DR, et al. Gaze-contingent motor channelling, haptic constraints and associated cognitive demand for robotic MIS. Med Image Anal. 2012;16(3):612–31.
24. Kitagawa M, Okamura AM, Bethea BT, et al. Analysis of suture manipulation forces for teleoperation with force feedback. In: Dohi T, Kikinis R, editors. Medical image computing and computer-assisted intervention. Berlin: Springer; 2002. p. 155–62.
25. Okamura AM. Methods for haptic feedback in teleoperated robot-assisted surgery. Ind Rob. 2004;31(6):499–508.
26. Mahvash M, Okamura A. Friction compensation for enhancing transparency of a teleoperator with compliant transmission. IEEE Trans Robot. 2007;23(6):1240–6.
27. Abbott JJ, Marayong P, Okamura AM. Haptic virtual fixtures for robot-assisted manipulation. In: Thrun S, Brooks R, Durrant-Whyte H, editors. Robotics research. Berlin: Springer; 2007. p. 49–64.
28. Reiley CE, Akinbiyi T, Burschka D, et al. Effects of visual force feedback on robot-assisted surgical task performance. J Thorac Cardiovasc Surg. 2008;135(1):196–202.
29. Masaya Kitagawa DD. Effect of sensory substitution on suture manipulation forces for surgical teleoperation. Stud Health Technol Inform. 2004;98:157.
30. Okamura AM. Haptic feedback in robot-assisted minimally invasive surgery. Curr Opin Urol. 2009;19(1):102.
31. Schneider O, Troccaz J. A six-degree-of-freedom passive arm with dynamic constraints (PADyC) for cardiac surgery application: preliminary experiments. Comput Aided Surg. 2001;6(6):340–51.
32. Davies B, Jakopec M, Harris SJ, et al. Active-constraint robotics for surgery. Proc IEEE. 2006;94(9):1696–704.
33. Lee S-L, Lerotic M, Vitiello V, et al. From medical images to minimally invasive intervention: computer assistance for robotic surgery. Comput Med Imaging Graph. 2010;34(1):33–45.
34. Ren J, Patel RV, Mcisaac KA, et al. Dynamic 3-D virtual fixtures for minimally invasive beating heart procedures. IEEE Trans Med Imaging. 2008;27(8):1061–70.
35. Kwok K-W, Mylonas GP, Sun LW, et al. Dynamic active constraints for hyper-redundant flexible robots. Med Image Comput Comput Assist Interv. 2009;12(Pt 1):410–7.
36. Kwok K-W, Vitiello V, Yang G-Z. Control of articulated snake robot under dynamic active constraints. In: Jiang T, Navab N, Pluim JPW, Viergever MA, editors. Medical image computing and computer-assisted intervention. Berlin: Springer; 2010. p. 229–36.
37. Molinero M B, Dagnino G, Liu J, et al. Haptic guidance for robot-assisted endovascular procedures: implementation and evaluation on surgical simulator. In: Proceedings of the 2019 IEEE/RSJ international conference on intelligent robots and systems (IROS). IEEE; 2019.
38. Kundrat D, Dagnino G, Kwok TM, et al. An MR-safe endovascular robotic platform: design, control, and ex-vivo evaluation. IEEE Trans Biomed Eng. 2021;68(10):3110–21.
39. Dagnino G, Georgilas I, Morad S, et al. Image-guided surgical robotic system for percutaneous reduction of joint fractures. Ann Biomed Eng. 2017;45(11):2648–62.
40. Dagnino G, Georgilas I, Morad S, et al. Intra-operative fiducial-based CT/fluoroscope image registration framework for image-guided robot-assisted joint fracture surgery. Int J Comput Assist Radiol Surg. 2017;12(8):1383–97.

Surgical Robotics

3

Contents

3.1 Introduction

This chapter provides an overview of the evolution of robotic surgery over the years, as well as the efforts undertaken in the integration of imaging, sensing, and robotics for improved human–robot interaction. It analyzes robotic platforms and technologies that have contributed to making robotic surgery a major area of innovation and development. Several exemplar platforms from both commercial and research organizations are reported here, categorized, and discussed. On the basis of the classification proposed by Bergeles et al. [1], we focus on different generations of robotic surgery. From one generation of robotic systems to the next, perception, decision, and action are becoming increasingly intertwined, resulting in improved control, dexterity and precision, and reduced invasiveness, access trauma, and tissue damage.

This chapter also focuses on the interaction between users and robotic systems regarding the tool and different levels of autonomy mapped to surgical platforms [2]. We cover five categories of tool motion: passive, teleoperated, semi-active, co-manipulated, and active [3]. In terms of the levels of autonomy, we discuss the range from no autonomy to robot-assistance, task autonomy, conditional autonomy, high

Y. Guo et al., *Medical Robotics*, Innovative Medical Devices,
https://doi.org/10.1007/978-981-99-7317-0_3

autonomy, all the way up to full autonomy [4]. Technologies for robotic surgery are also described, including different imaging modalities (both preoperative and intraoperative, e.g., fluoroscopy, CT, MRI, etc.) and sensing technologies, and their integration in the control architecture of a robotic platform to provide enhanced navigation (visual and haptic guidance).

3.2 Evolution Trends of Surgical Robots

This section follows the evolution of surgical robots with decreasing invasiveness and collateral tissue damage but increasing surgical dexterity. It mostly includes systems that have been commercialized or novel research systems with extensive in vivo validation, highlighting their clinical impact. Figure 3.1 provides a timeline of surgical robots, showing key milestones in robotic surgery and computer-assisted intervention, as well as the evolution of robotic platforms throughout different generations. Typical examples are summarized in Table 3.1. This section is not intended to provide an exhaustive taxonomy of research publications; instead, we refer the readers to existing reviews on medical robotics [1, 2, 5, 11, 16, 19–37].

3.2.1 Neurosurgery and Orthopedics

As mentioned in the previous chapter, due to the well-defined and rigid nature of structures involved in orthopedics surgery as well as stereotaxic neurosurgery (e.g., bones), the first generation of surgical robots was used in these fields. This makes it easier to register the robotic system with the patient and maintain the registration during the entire surgery to allow for real-time intraoperative navigation, tracking, and closed-loop vision-based robot control [2]. These solutions primarily address the lack of dexterity in MIS [1] by focusing on improving surgical accuracy rather than just providing the surgeon with visual or haptic guidance.

In the first application of a robotic system in neurosurgery, Kwoh et al. [38] used the PUMA 200 (Unimation, Danbury, USA), an industrial robotic manipulator, to position a mechanical guide used by the surgeon to introduce a needle and perform a brain biopsy. This robotic system was successfully tested on a patient in April 1985.

Since then, the use of adapted industrial robots in neurosurgery [39] has gradually shifted toward bespoke robotic systems developed specifically for clinical tasks. The Neuromate (Renishaw, New Mills, UK) is one of the first neurosurgical robots to be accepted by the FDA in the United States and to obtain CE certification in Europe. This system uses a 5-DoF image-guided semi-active robot to place surgical tools (such as needles) precisely and accurately along predetermined paths. It is used for a variety of neurosurgery operations, such as electrode implantation, biopsy, and neuroendoscopy. The software of the robot enables the intraoperative registration of preoperative 3D (CT, MRI) and intraoperative (X-ray, US) [6] and automatically positions the surgical tool holder using preoperative planning. Moreover, the Neuromate can operate in a frameless mode, using an implantable base mounted on the patient to link fiducial markers from CT and MRI

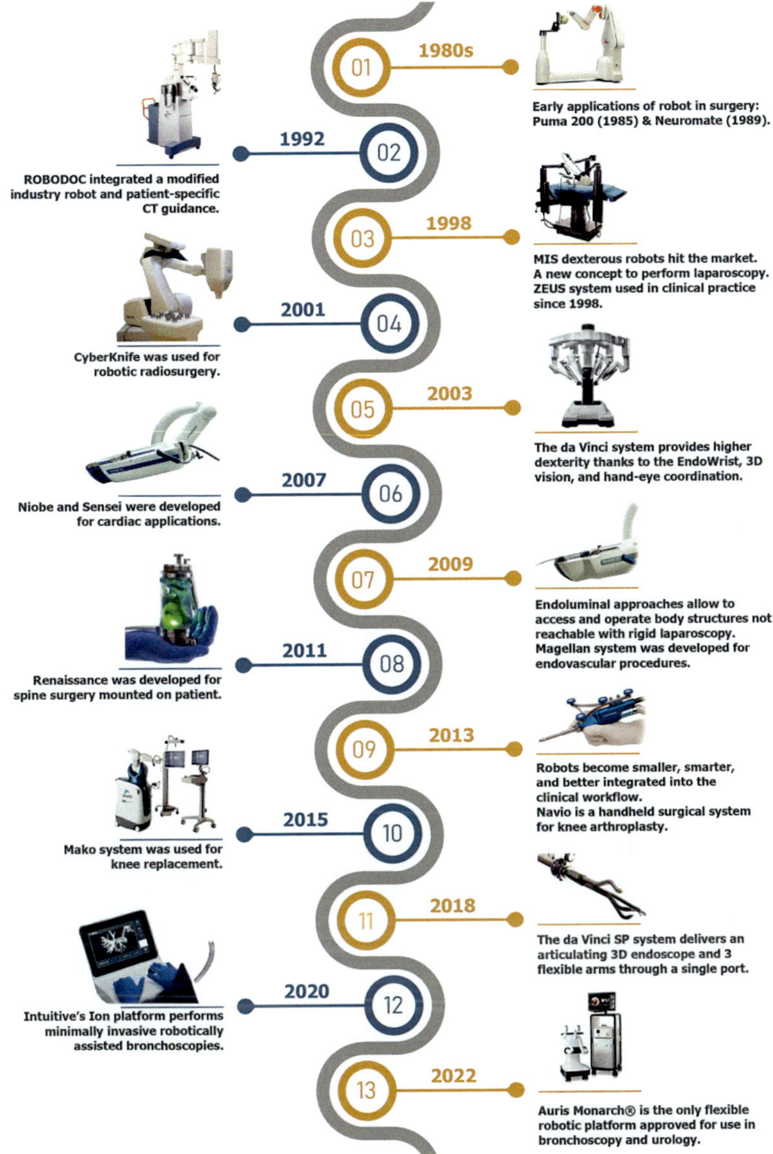

Fig. 3.1 Timeline of surgical robots. Since the first application of a robot in surgery in 1985, a growing number of robotic surgical platforms have been developed and applied to several clinical specializations. From bulky industrial arms adapted to be used in clinical applications—typical of the infancy of robotic surgery—robotic platforms have been bespoke designed to facilitate clinical usability and have become smaller and smarter. This figure reports key milestones in robotics surgery (only commercial platforms) of the last 40 years. neuromateNeuro-mate, Renishaw, © 2023; ROBODOC (CC BY 4.0); ZEUS/AESOP, © Computer Motion; CyberKnife (CC BY 2.0); da Vinci/da Vinci SP/Ion, Intuitive Surgical Inc., © 2023; Sensei and Niobe (adapted with Springer Nature permission from [5]); Mazor Robotics Renaissance, Mazor Robotics; Navio, Smith+&Nephew, © 2023; Mako, Stryiker, © 2023; Monarch, Johnson+&Johnson MedTthech, © 2023

Table 3.1 Overview of exemplary medical robots commercially available

Type	Robotic platforms	Company	Clinical application	Vision	Sensing	Level of automation	Ref.
Stereotaxic neurosurgery and orthopedics	Neuromate	Renishaw PLC (UK)	Neurosurgery	3D	No	Semi-active (parallel)	[6]
	ROBODOC	Curexo Technology (USA)	Orthopedics	3D	Force	Active	[7]
	Acrobot	Stryker (USA)	Orthopedics	3D	Force	Semi-active (parallel)	[8]
	NAVIO	Smith&Nephew (UK)	Orthopedics	Infrared guidance	No	Semi-active (serial)	[9]
	Mako	Stryker (USA)	Orthopedics	3D	Force	Semi-active (parallel)	[10]
	Renaissance	Mazor Robotics (Israel)	Spine surgery	3D	No	Semi-active (parallel)	[11]
	CyberKnife	Accuray (USA)	Radiation therapy	3D	No	Active	[12]
Robotic laparoscopy and flexible robotics	ZEUS/AESOP	Computer Motion (USA)	Laparoscopy	2D	No	Teleoperated	[13]
	da Vinci	Intuitive Surgical Inc. (USA)	Laparoscopy	3D	No	Teleoperated	[14]
	Niobe	Stereotaxis (USA)	Vascular surgery	3D	No	Teleoperated	[15]
	Sensei	Hansen Medical (now Auris) (USA)	Vascular surgery	3D	Force	Teleoperated	[16]
	Magellan	Hansen Medical (now Auris) (USA)	Vascular surgery	2D	No	Teleoperated	[16]
	CorPath GRX	Siemens Healthineers (Germany)	Vascular surgery	2D	No	Teleoperated	[17]
	Monarch	Johnson & Johnson (USA)	Bronchoscopy/ urology	3D	No	Teleoperated	[18]
Untethered microrobotics	PillCam	Medtronic (USA)	Capsule endoscopy	2D	n/a	Passive	[19]
	EndoCapsule	Olympus (Japan)	Capsule endoscopy	2D	n/a	Passive	[19]

images into patient coordinates [21]. In a frame-based configuration, the system achieves a positioning accuracy of 0.86 mm, while in a frameless configuration, it achieves an accuracy of 1.95 mm [6]. Systems like neuroArm [40] emphasize the clinical need for smaller platforms that can be seamlessly integrated into the operating room's surgical flow. Novel technologies aiming at reducing the component size of the robots will allow for this integration. For example, only one robotic arm could fit inside the MRI when the first neuroArm was launched. By the second generation, functionality had significantly increased by fitting two arms into the scanner [41].

Many other robotic platforms were created to work under MR imaging, such as the stereotactic MR-compatible robots that may be installed outside the magnet [42] developed by the Brigham and Women's Hospital in Boston, Massachusetts, and the Surgical Assist Technology Group in Tsukuba, Japan. The continual quest for better imaging in the field of neurosurgery explains the motivation to combine robotics with MRI's greater depiction of soft tissue contrast.

Newer needle-insertion robots are miniaturized to be mountable on the skull and spine of the patients [11, 43]. The Mazor Robotics Renaissance (Mazor Robotics, Caesarea, Israel) is a semi-active surgical robot that can be mounted directly onto a patient to perform spine surgery. To follow the patient's motion and make integration in the operating room easier, the robot is positioned directly on the patient's spine. Based on preoperative CT planning, the Renaissance robot precisely guides the surgeon to place tools and implants in the patient's spine [44].

Another commercially available frameless robot is the CyberKnife (Accuray Inc., Sunnyvalve, USA), a radiotherapy robotic system used to treat cranial and spinal tumors as well as other cancers like pancreatic and liver cancers. Its integrated imaging system has the ability to autonomously detect and compensate for patients' and organs' motion [12] in order to provide the greatest radiation dose to the tumor while protecting surrounding healthy organs and tissues. With more than 100,000 patients treated globally [45], this system is considered a standard for radiotherapy. Neurosurgical and orthopedic surgical robots both underwent simultaneous development. ROBODOC (Curexo Technology, Fremont, USA) [46] was the first commercial surgical robot for orthopedics, specifically for total hip replacement. A CT image of the patient's anatomy is taken for preoperative planning in order to precisely cut a hollow in the femur and install the replacement implant. Fiducials (pins) that were inserted into the bone prior to the CT scan are visible in the planning data and touched by the robot prior to the surgery to transfer the plan to the patient. ROBODOC is completely autonomous and operates under the surgeon's monitoring that can make adjustments as necessary. For safety considerations, it mounts a 6-axis load cell, which pioneered the use of force sensing in robotic surgery [18]. The system reached the market in 1994, commercialized by Integrated Surgical Systems (Sacramento, USA). The UK counterpart for total knee replacement, called Acrobot, was created by Davies et al. at Imperial College London [8]. It utilizes a preoperative CT scan of the patient to create the surgical plan. Acrobot cooperates synergistically with the surgeon to complete the operation rather than performing it autonomously [47]. Active constraints are generated by the planning software to direct the surgeon during milling operations, ensuring that the robot only moves in designated, permissible zones [48]. A 6-DOF force sensor is mounted on the robot to close the control of the system. Another semi-active robotic system for knee replacement is the Mako system (Stryker, Kalamazoo, USA). Similar to Acrobot, Mako creates a model of the patient's knee using preoperative CT images in order to arrange the procedure beforehand. With the use of image registration, the surgeon is able to control the burr while viewing a 3D model of the knee during surgery. The technology limits the burr's workspace by generating no-fly zones to prevent damaging the bone outside of the designated locations and by providing both haptic and auditory guidance [10]. As mentioned in the previous chapter, smaller-scale frameless systems were created as a result of the growing need for custom-designed, more manageable, and clinically usable robotic systems that could be quickly integrated into the surgical workflow. The Navio, for instance, is a handheld robotic driller for knee arthroplasty by Smith & Nephew, UK. Through the use of an infrared camera and optical instruments, Navio continuously tracks the patient's anatomy as well as the handheld robotic device [9]. With this methodology, preoperative CT scans and intraoperative registration are not required. By moving the tracked optical probe over the anatomy to construct a physical map of it, a 3D model of the knee is produced. The Navio uses a speed/exposure control safeguard that is delivered using the handheld robotized tool, allowing the excision of bone layers that have been identified by the surgeon.

Robotic surgical systems with a focus on fracture surgery have been developed in addition to arthroplasty applications [49–51]. For instance, Dogramadzi et al. created the *Robot-Assisted Fracture Surgery* (RAFS) surgical system, a robotic platform to reduce knee fractures [51–54]. Based on preoperative planning, RAFS is an active robotic system that provides percutaneous reduction of distal femur fractures. To virtually reduce the fracture before surgery, the surgeon can manipulate CT-generated 3D bone models of a specific fracture. The preoperative planning is registered with the patient in the operating room, and the robot completes the physical reduction while the surgeon can make adjustments as necessary. RAFS tracks both the patient's anatomy and the robotic manipulators to offer real-time intraoperative 3D navigation, and force sensing is implemented in the control loop for safety purposes. The system was tested on human cadavers in 2016 [51]. The rigid nature of bones makes the registration between robotic systems and patients' images easy and consistent, thus the preplanning of robot trajectories possible. However, as seen, there are a number of challenges that must be taken into consideration while performing surgical procedures on soft tissues. Limitations include the difficulty of tracking deformable anatomy and the possibility of providing reliable force and visual guidance. The next-generation surgical robots, which are based on synergistic cooperation between the robot and the surgeon, integration of various imaging modalities, and increased dexterity in manipulating soft tissue in a constrained operating space, have the goal of overcoming such limitations.

3.2.2 Robotic Laparoscopy and Flexible Robots for Endoluminal Interventions

The category of medical robotics that is probably the most developed and certainly the most profitable is robotic laparoscopy [55]. Initial robotic systems in this category were basically robotic arms that could manipulate the camera endoscope to do away with the need for further human assistants. The first example is AESOP, the first FDA-approved robotic surgical device that holds and moves the video endoscope to various locations using voice control and resembles the form and function of a human arm [56]. The first surgical robots for minimally invasive applications started to appear in the early 1990s. PROBOT [57] was a modified version of the industrial robot PUMA 560 with a safety frame to restrict the arm's workspace. It was created for prostatectomy. The ZEUS platform (Computer Motion, USA) [13] was created with the idea of performing laparoscopic procedures using several robotic arms that may be teleoperated from a remote station. Tremor filtering and motion scaling are features of the ZEUS robotic arms, which mimic surgeon movements and increase surgical accuracy. It was used in the well-known transatlantic robot-assisted cholecystectomy (by Marescaux et al., with the patient in Strasbourg, France, and the surgeons in New York [58]) before being withdrawn from the market in favor of the da Vinci system. The da Vinci robot, probably the most famous surgical robotic platform on the market, is widely used in a variety of surgical procedures, including prostatectomy, cholecystectomy, fundoplication, and colorectal surgery. The surgeon grasps two master controls below the display that offers an immersive 3D visualization of the surgical field, restoring hand-eye coordination. The stereo vision provided by the 3D endoscope allows the restoration of the sense of depth that is missing in traditional laparoscopy. The surgeon manipulates the anatomy using the EndoWrist instruments (e.g., for manipulating, suturing, clamping, etc.) with 7-DoF, something that is not achievable with normal laparoscopy.

Despite these advantages, da Vinci does not provide haptic feedback. In the past decade, the da Vinci robot has technically evolved and commercially grown (data according to the company's annual report 2021, see https://isrg.gcs-web.com/). Approximately 6800 units have been used, and more than 150 different instruments have been released for the da Vinci, resulting in more than 1.5 million procedures being completed. These data were further growing in 2022 with an expected growth rate of +14% (a bit less than the pre-pandemic trend of +18% due to the impact that COVID-19 had, and is still having, on surgical procedures rate). Parallel to this, the initial patents that had granted Intuitive Surgical a monopoly position in robotic laparoscopic surgery started to lapse, leading a number of significant medical equipment companies to initiate initiatives to create their own robots that are gradually introduced into the market [55].

Academic research developed concurrently with commercial advancements on two different fronts: (1) enhancing surgeons' capabilities and (2) reducing the invasiveness of the procedures. On the first front, the advent of open platform robots for research purposes, the beginnings of surgical automation development, and ongoing efforts to incorporate force sensing into laparoscopic equipment are the main subtopics. On the second front, single-port systems have drawn the greatest attention, including the da Vinci SP, a recently released commercial device from Intuitive [55]. As explained in the previous chapters, miniaturized flexible robots represent a promising technology that could improve MIS through transluminal and/or endoluminal procedures (e.g., no need for skin incisions to access internal anatomy, deeper access along tortuous anatomical passages, as illustrated in Fig. 3.2). For example, the i-Snake—a snake-like tendon-driven robot with full retroflection capabilities developed by Yang and colleagues—allows exploration of a large area of the anatomy through NOTES without requiring laparoscopic-style external manipulation [63].

Another robotic platform, the Micro-IGES, was created again by Yang et al. [60] with the goal of enhancing the precision and accuracy of endoluminal tasks through integrated sensing, probe-based microscopy, and robot-assisted intraoperative guidance.

The platforms mentioned above can access a number of anatomical locations in the human body but, due to larger dimensions, are not able to operate in restricted areas such as vessels, kidneys, or brain. As a result, concentric tube robots and steerable catheters with a few millimeters in diameter have been created. In endovascular procedures, catheters are utilized to move through the vasculature, get to the desired anatomy, and carry out the clinical procedure, such as stenting, ablation, embolization, and device delivery [64]. Robotic steerable-catheter technology is becoming more popular due to the difficult maneuverability of catheters, which may result in serious damage to the vessels. Benefits include increased stability and precision, access to tortuous and challenging anatomy, and decreased radiation exposure for both the patient and the operator. Robotic platforms that are commercially available—such as the Hansen Medical's Sensei X2 and the Magellan—are used for endovascular and EP applications, respectively [16]. These platforms feature tendon-driven steerable catheters that are teleoperated by the operator seated at a remote console via joystick and buttons. The Sensei X2 offers the integration of 3D guidance through the compatible EnSite Precision (St. Jude Medical, Saint Paul, USA) or CARTO3 (Biosense Webster, Brussels, Belgium) 3D mapping systems. The Magellan system still depends on 2D fluoroscopic imaging for guidance.

Another teleoperated commercial platform utilized in EP applications is called Niobe (Stereotaxis, St. Louis, USA) [15], which uses a magnetic field created by two permanent magnets to control the orientation of specially built EP catheters and guidewires using a mouse or joystick at the control station. The CARTO3 system is integrated to enable 3D navigation, minimizing the patient's exposure to X-rays. Additionally, because the control station is located outside the operating room, the operator is not exposed to X-ray radiation.

Other emerging robotic platforms for endovascular intervention include the CorPath GRX (Siemens Healthineers, Erlangen, Germany) and the R-One (Robocath, Rouen, France) used in endovascular applications. Researchers at Imperial College London have developed an MR-safe robotic platform for endovascular intervention that features enhanced instrument maneuverability, multimodal image guidance (standard fluoroscopy and MRI), and vision-based haptic feedback. After benchtop studies with end-users, the system was successfully tested on in vivo animals [61, 65–67].

The steerable catheter robots' inability to exert strong forces is one of their key drawbacks. Concentric tube robots have the necessary flexibility to navigate

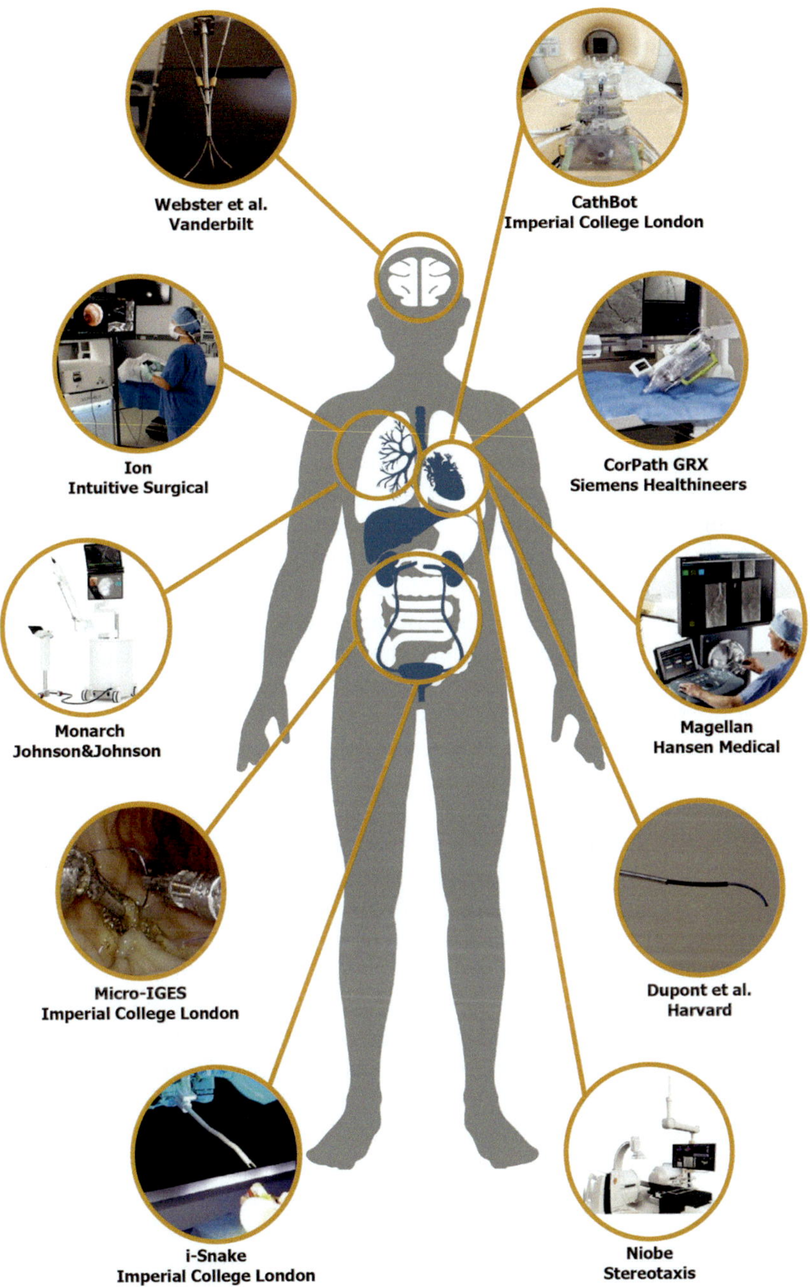

Fig. 3.2 Exemplary robots for endoluminal applications. Robot developed by Webster et al. (adapted with SAGE permission from [59]); Ion, Intuitive Surgical Inc., © 2023; Monarch, Johnson&Johnson MedTech, © 2023; Micro-IGES (adapted with IEEE permission from [60]); i-Snake (adapted with IEEE permission from [1]); CathBot (adapted from [61] (CC BY 4.0)); CorPath GRX, Siemens Healthineers, © 2023; Magellan and Niobe (adapted with Springer Nature permission from [16]); Robot developed by Dupont et al. (adapted with AAAS permission from [62])

complex anatomy while offering increased stiffness. They are made up of nested sets of pre-curved elastic tubes that bend and deform when they are translated and rotated with respect to one another. Around 2005, research teams led by Sears and Dupont [68], Webster [69], and Furusho et al. [70] pioneered this research area, which is now applicable to a variety of surgical applications such as cardiology and ENT. Additionally, steerable catheter-based commercial systems for minimally invasive biopsies through natural orifices have just lately been introduced. For example, the Ion system by Intuitive Surgical and the Monarch system by Auris Healthcare employ dexterous catheter articulation to perform peripheral lung biopsies, which would otherwise be highly challenging.

3.2.3 Untethered Microrobots

Although flexible robots are promising for the future of MIS, newer enabling technologies are paving the way toward the next generation of surgical robots. Wireless capsule endoscopes and microrobots promise enhanced diagnostic and therapeutic capabilities as well as potentially unlimited intracorporeal navigation [19]. Given Imaging (Yokneam Illit, Israel—now Medtronic) introduced PillCam in 2001—a wireless capsule that can inspect the gastrointestinal tract in a minimally invasive way. The possibility of using a "pill" that can navigate the colon and capture images from deep inside revolutionized gastrointestinal endoscopy and gave rise to a brand-new area of study called medical capsule robots [55]. Capsule robots are small devices (11 mm in diameter and 26 mm in length) that can be swallowed to navigate the GI system by peristalsis (in around 8–10 h) in order to carry out image-based diagnosis. Since the introduction of PillCam, several other devices have been launched, such as the EndoCapsule (Olympus, Japan) [19]. Please refer to the comprehensive review by Valdastri et al. [19].

Despite the clear benefit of increased comfort for the patient with respect to standard endoscopy, capsule endoscopes present a number of technical and clinical limitations. These include: (1) no active controllability that prevents a camera's atypical movement (such as moving closer to a suspicious lesion); (2) sub-optimal tissue interaction that prevents the collection of biopsy; and (3) restricted field of view that could lead to false-negative diagnoses. There have been numerous studies on the actuation for capsule active locomotion, with both onboard and external locomotion strategies proposed. Dario [71] and Kim [72] presented bio-inspired onboard locomotion systems, but these actuation schemes have significant power consumption, limited functioning time, and low controllability [19]. These problems have been attempted to be solved using external locomotion methods. Here, either electro-magnets or permanent magnets are used to produce a strong magnetic field close to the patient in order to control the capsule inside [73, 74]. In addition, capsule endoscopes may conduct biopsies utilizing a variety of sample methods, including magnetic-field-actuated blades [75], thermosensitive tissue-cutting razors [76], and screw-type capsules that can penetrate soft tissue [74]. This opens the door for additional sampling methods.

In the coming years, smart control of untethered microrobots may offer unprecedented diagnostic and therapeutic capabilities when combined with multimodal imaging (e.g., multi-spectral, autofluorescence, and micro-ultrasound). Advantages in energy storage or wireless power transfer are also needed [55]. It is envisioned that this will allow microrobots to become essential tools for early-stage detection and precision treatment of diseases [1].

3.3 Technologies for Robotic Surgery

The previous section has provided an overview of the evolution of robotic surgery, introducing the various generations of surgical robots, reporting commercial and emerging platforms, and highlighting their clinical impact and innovation.

Before looking ahead and discussing the unmet demands and future challenges, it is important to examine the current state-of-the-art underpinning technologies for robotic surgery (see Fig. 3.3).

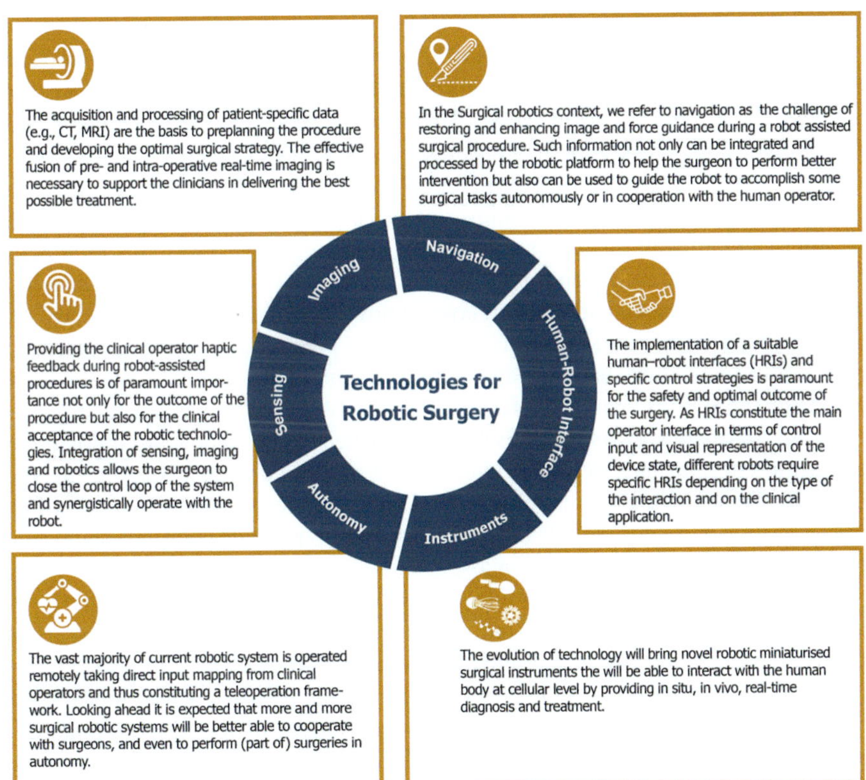

Fig. 3.3 Underpinning technologies for robotic surgery, including imaging, sensing, autonomy, instruments, navigation, and human–machine interfaces

3.3.1 Human–Robot Interaction and Levels of Autonomy

As seen in the previous section, surgical robots are used to perform a wide range of surgical tasks, and the required technology has evolved.

This has made it possible for robots to function accurately in constrained spaces with little harm to soft tissue and even to be implanted inside of patients or taken internally to perform intracorporeal procedures and/or find pathologies [2]. The development of surgical robots includes not only changes in size and architecture but also improvements in safety features and cooperative behavior with the surgical team. The use of appropriate HRIs and targeted control measures is crucial for the safety and successful completion of the procedure. Troccaz et al. categorized surgical robots based on how the user and the robotic system interact with tool motion [3]:

1. Active robots are those that autonomously execute a preplanned motion.
2. Passive robots are unactuated and manually driven.
3. Semi-active (e.g., cooperated) robots employ constrained motion.
4. Teleoperated robots involve a tool held by the robot and remotely controlled by the human.

As *Human–Machine Interfaces* (HMIs) constitute the main operator interface in terms of control input and visual representation of the device state, it is clear that different robots require specific HMIs depending on the type of the interaction and on the clinical application. In the last decade, various HMI concepts were proposed in endoluminal robotics. Many research platforms and commercial devices still use conventional joysticks (one to multiple degrees of freedom), which are mapped to the robot end-effector displacement, feeding, rotating, or bending. This limitation has been addressed in research by different strategies: (1) design of task-specific HMIs and (2) abstraction of the input layer to novel concepts and feedback cues. As an example, a highly customized HMIs has been presented for endovascular surgery, replicating clinical handling and motion patterns of conventional catheters and guidewires [65]. This approach has been well received by senior vascular surgeons due to its transparency. Notably, it is further expected to reduce operator training for a transition from manual to robotic interventions as motion input is mapped equivalently to manual procedures. Similarly, flexible electronic circuits are proposed for the realization of customized HMIs to enhance user control and feedback, for example, the circuits of soft robots for endoscopy.

The concept of robot autonomy is strictly linked to HRI. The vast majority of current robotic systems are operated remotely, taking direct input mapping from clinical operators and thus constituting a teleoperation framework (i.e., a setup with HMIs and remote robotic manipulator). To the present day, this is the clinical gold standard in robotic surgery and reflects the lowest autonomy level according to the taxonomy, with six independent autonomy levels in total presented in Yang et al. [4]. This definition comprises no autonomy (level 0) with robotic control based on direct operator input to fully autonomous execution and completion of the robotic task without human interaction (level 5). Looking ahead, it is expected that surgical robotic systems will increasingly be better able to cooperate with surgeons and even to perform (part of) surgeries in autonomy. Currently, only partial automation, i.e., fully predictable device behaviors, of workflow phases is realized in commercial endoluminal devices; i.e., sequences of motion primitives are executed automatically to support teleoperation. As an example, the CorPath GRX platform (Siemens Healthineers, Erlangen, Germany) features partial procedural automation of guidewire manipulation (e.g., spin to cross lesions), mimicking motion patterns from manual instrument handling. Studies on conditional approaches (autonomy level 3) using a robotic platform in combination with generative adversarial imitation learning have demonstrated feasibility and enhanced cannulation results [77]. In terms of human cooperation, (partial) autonomy enables enhanced support of the surgeon in certain situations, e.g., navigating through challenging anatomy. However, there is a lack of clinical studies involving autonomous behavior with the exception of robotic laparoscopic surgery [78]. In Saeidi et al. [79], in vivo autonomous surgery for intestinal anastomosis on porcine models using a setup of two robotic arms with suturing device and endoscopic vision has been presented.

The use of autonomy in surgical robots is still quite limited, despite the fact that the development of autonomous driving capabilities has arguably been one of the hottest topics in robotics over the past decade [55]. To give the robot the ability to create and modify its plans and motions based on real-time information, it is necessary to better integrate imaging and sensing. Along with technological difficulties, there are still legal, ethical, and regulatory issues that need to be handled. As suggested by Dupont et al. [55], "an evolutionary trend toward progressive automation will provide time for the necessary technological developments in algorithms and sensors while allowing stakeholders time to progressively construct an appropriate regulatory and legal framework." It appears clear that this can be achieved only through a deep collaboration between engineers, clinicians, regulators, investors, and the business community.

3.3.2 Computer-Assisted Intervention: Integrating Imaging and Sensing

New surgical robotic systems should be able to work alongside surgeons, giving them superhuman dexterity as well as integrated real-time intraoperative image guiding, sensing, and decision-making. The surgeon will be able to close the system's control loop and work in concert with the robot thanks to information gathered through sight and sense.

The acquisition and processing of patient-specific data (e.g., CT, MRI) are the basis for preplanning the procedure and developing the optimal surgical strategy. In order to support the clinical team in providing the best care and achieving cost-effective outcomes, it is essential that preoperative planning, intraoperative real-time imaging, sensing, and robotic assistance are effectively combined [2]. Computer-assisted intervention's original purpose was to help doctors carry out effective and secure diagnostic or therapeutic procedures. To support the decision-making and action-taking processes, it is crucial to collect patient data and information about the procedure being performed. The creation of specific sensors and data processing could be necessary during this stage.

It is critical that clinicians combine patient-specific data with medical knowledge, such as the phase of a surgical procedure, anatomical atlases, or organ shapes. However, this step is frequently done mentally and qualitatively. One of the main objectives is to combine all the data into a single quantitative model to inform the decision-making (e.g., in radiotherapy, determining the radiation dose to a tumor while preserving the surrounding healthy tissues). Additionally, preplanning can be done through procedural simulation, for instance, by simulating the interactions between instruments and organs. However, this is very challenging, as target organs move and intraoperative information may have to be acquired to update or replan a strategy accordingly so that guiding systems can execute the planned action on the patient.

3.3.3 Surgical Navigation and Control

The introduction of robotics, in conjunction with computer assistance, has brought a tremendous benefit in terms of superhuman dexterity and precision. However, due to the indirect visualization of the surgical site during robot-assisted procedures as well as the removal of the surgeon's hands from the tissues being manipulated, image and force guidance are necessary to improve the accuracy and safety of these procedures. Here, we refer to the challenges of restoring and enhancing image and force guidance as "Surgical Navigation" (see Fig. 3.4). As already mentioned above, such information can be integrated and processed by the robotic platform to help the surgeon perform better intervention but can also be used to guide the robot to accomplish some surgical tasks autonomously or in cooperation with the human operator.

Volumetric preoperative imaging (e.g., CT, MRI) is commonly used for diagnostic purposes and used to preplan the surgical procedure. While these imaging modalities provide accurate 3D information necessary to perform the diagnosis and planning, they have limited temporal capabilities; i.e., it takes time to acquire the data. This limitation, together with logistic constraints (they need big and appropriately shielded rooms), makes these image modalities not yet suited to be directly used intraoperatively where the temporal resolution is of paramount importance. Contrary to preoperative imaging, however, real-time intraoperative data collection is constrained. As previously indicated, US imaging is reasonably priced, accessible at most hospitals, and useful for guiding and identifying soft tissue during minimally invasive surgery. Although X-ray fluoroscopy is frequently utilized for intravascular applications, soft tissues are not visible to the operator without the addition of iodine contrast. Good soft tissue contrast can be achieved using real-time MRI guiding, but only a few 2D pictures can be obtained to achieve the necessary temporal resolution, and MR-safe devices must be used for any interventions inside an MR scanner.

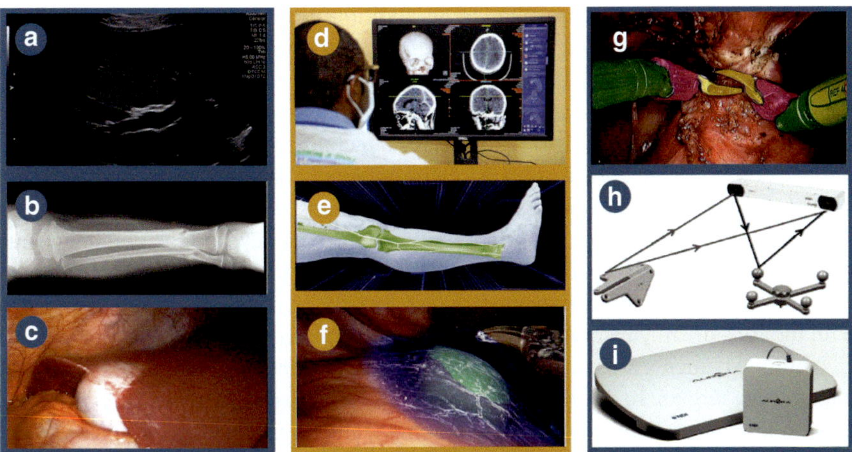

Fig. 3.4 Surgical navigation. On the left (**a–c**) are three types of standard imaging commonly used for intraoperative guidance during surgery: ultrasounds (**a**), fluoroscopy (**b**), and video laparoscopy (**c**). The mid column (**d–f**) shows enhanced surgical navigation: 3D preoperative imaging can be registered to intraoperative imaging modalities to enhance 3D visual navigation (**f**) and enable virtual and augmented reality (**e, f**) as well as robotic assistance and haptic guidance. In the context of surgical navigation, in addition to knowing the position of the anatomy during the procedure, one fundamental requirement is to detect and track the location and trajectory of the robotics end-effectors. This can be done via dedicated tracking software (**g**) or using devices such as optical (**h**) and electromagnetic (**i**) trackers. Images **a–g** are publicly available on Wikimedia Commons and Creative Commons (CC BY 4.0); images **h** and **i**, NDI, © 2023

A number of MR-compatible robotic systems have already been developed [65, 80, 81]. For example, Yang and colleagues [65, 66] investigated the feasibility of an MR-compatible robot that can be used in various endovascular procedures. It is anticipated that more MR-compatible robots will be developed. However, a combination of intraoperative and preoperative data is still required for navigation, as well as their registration to the intraoperative workspace. Registration between multiple imaging modalities, scans, and times is also needed [82–84]. The registration process gains another dimension when a 3D model of the anatomy is used. We have seen that it is still difficult to track tissue deformation during surgery [34]. Dynamic shape instantiation [85] makes use of preoperative 3D models and adapts them to the surgical scene using limited intraoperative images, resulting in a fast and not computationally expensive registration.

Computer vision methods to create 3D surfaces directly from the surgical video are another method for 3D deformation modeling for intraoperative guidance [86]. Through augmented reality, preoperative or intraoperative data can be superimposed into the exposed surgical perspective, as opposed to traditionally reviewing preoperative data before an operation or displaying it alongside the preoperative scene. The optimal way to integrate and convey preoperative and intraoperative data into the surgical scene without disrupting the surgical workflow has been the subject of extensive research [5].

In the context of surgical robotics, in addition to knowing the position of the anatomy during the procedure, one fundamental requirement is to detect and track the location and trajectory of the robotics end-effectors. Surgical robotic systems conventionally use external measurement devices that track sensors that are mounted on the robot end-effectors in real time. Several technologies have been used, including various types of optical sensors, electromagnetic sensors, ultrasonic sensors, and even GPS-based technology [87]. Requirements of surgical position sensors include position and orientation accuracy, update frequency, and the number of targets simultaneously trackable. It is usually necessary to determine the position of the tracked device in three, five, or six DoFs, i.e., the (x,y,z) spatial location together with the roll–pitch–yaw orientations relative to a reference.

Multiple cameras are used by *optical position sensors* to pinpoint the location of one or more targets. In the beginning, systems used reflective markers applied to the patient that were then manually or automatically digitalized in various camera angles. The majority of contemporary systems, like the Polaris (NDI, Canada), utilize 2D *Charge Coupled Device* (CCD) arrays with excellent resolution that are filtered to only allow intense infrared light in a certain limited frequency band to be seen by the cameras. Optical technologies have also been employed in robotic surgical interventions for a very long time [53]. They can be more advantageous than position monitoring based solely on encoders and are simple to add to the system. All optical systems present the line-of-sight problem, which means that a continuous, unobstructed path must be kept between the cameras and the instrument's targets. In surgical settings, this can occasionally be difficult and inconvenient. The transmitter, or field generator, is the main component of *Electromagnetic* (EM) tracking systems. The EM field created by the emitter coils in the field generator is picked up by sensors. The position sensor picks up the current that is induced by this field in the receiving coil. The position of the sensor can be determined using factors like the intensity or phase of the receiver current. In most EM systems, a single sensor coil provides at least 5-DoF. This means that it is possible to know the end effector's (x, y, z) position as well as its pitch-yaw orientation. Metal and ferromagnetic materials distort the magnetic field and are typically not suitable to be used with EM systems. EM systems do not suffer from line-of-sight problems, which—together with their small size—represent an advantage over optical technologies. Various devices, such as needles, catheters, and even vascular guidewires, can mount such tiny sensors. The Aurora (NDI, Canada) is one exemplary EM tracking system.

Impedance systems are used in the field of electrophysiological mapping and ablation. The measurements are made using the same catheters used for the cardiac electrical measurements, making them suitable for intracorporal measurement. The mechanisms are also out of line of sight and unaffected by environmental metal contamination. For instance, Biosense Webster's CARTO3 uses an impedance-based technology, but it is combined with their EM system to calibrate the environment in real time, enhancing the accuracy. This tracking system is employed along with robotics platforms such as Stereotaxis "Epoch" and the and Hansen "Sensei" to navigate robotically driven catheters. However, the tracking accuracy that can be achieved with this technology is limited.

We have discussed that in order to give surgeons the necessary perceptual information for navigation and the best use of force during image-guided robotic surgery, it is crucial to include haptic feedback in the robot control interface. Active constraints were the main focus of early haptic rendering research, with the aforementioned Acrobot surgical system as a prominent example [8]. When the cutter approaches the predetermined banned region, the active constraint control device gradually increases the haptic stiffness of the surgeon's hand via the handle. Virtual fixtures work on the principle of a ruler guiding a pen, which lessens the stress on some human sensory modalities when processing the remote-control operation. The ability to provide force feedback to human operators and assess tissue handling proficiency could be enabled by knowledge of interaction forces during teleoperated robot-assisted surgery. Direct force sensing at the end-effector is difficult, though, because it requires biocompatible and sterile sensors. Dagnino et al. [67] developed a vision-based haptic guidance framework that was integrated into robot-assisted endovascular intervention. Dynamic active constraints are generated by tracking via image processing the relative position of vascular instruments and the vasculature. The closer the instruments are to the vessel wall, the higher the friction will be rendered at the master robot. The goal is to guide the operator during the procedure while avoiding potentially harmful peak-force impacts between the instruments and the vessel walls. Recently, Okamura et al. [88] presented a force estimation neural network that uses RGB images and robot state as inputs to estimate forces during robot-assisted minimally invasive surgery. This is the first combined vision and state network that uses both position and force-torque state estimates as inputs to complement vision inputs.

3.4 What the Future Holds: Micro-Nano Robotics for Surgery

As analyzed in the previous sections of this chapter, robotic surgical platforms have the benefit of increasing dexterity, manipulation, and navigation (imaging and sensing) capabilities of the clinical team. In particular, the confluence and advances of diverse technologies (e.g., motors, control theory, materials, medical imaging) have enabled a revolution in surgical applications of robotic technologies [89].

However, reaching and treating with surgical platforms small and early lesions located in regions of the human body difficult to access still presents some significant technological obstacles, such as mechanical parts still quite large and not flexible. The development of miniaturized, adaptable robots with dimensions of a few micrometers will pave the way for new procedures that can reach the cellular level and provide localized diagnosis and treatment with greater accuracy and efficiency. In this section, key challenges and future directions of micro-nano robotics for surgery are summarized. Readers are referred to Li et al. [89] for an updated and detailed overview of this evolving field.

Recent advances in nanotechnology and materials are driving the development of novel micro-nano robots [89]. However, achieving a successful translation toward wider patient use continues to be a major challenge due to safety issues and the complexity of navigating and interacting with the human body [90].

As conventional power supply components and batteries are not possible at these micro- and nano-scales, locomotion is the first obstacle for the miniaturization of robots, and innovative designs are therefore necessary to satisfy the demanding powering and movement requirements. Micro/nano robots, for instance, can run on chemically fueled motors that transform locally provided fuels into force and motion, or they can use externally powered motors that move by using magnetic and ultrasonic energies [89].

Recent advances in micro- and nanorobots have shown considerable promise for using these tiny devices for precision surgery (see Fig. 3.5). For example, micro- and nanorobotic tools, such as nanodrillers, microgrippers, or microbullets, offer unique capabilities for early and targeted intervention.

For precise surgery, nanodrillers can be used to enter biological tissues. These tiny robots can perform tasks at the cellular level via the body's smallest capillaries [89]. Microgrippers can interact with tissues and cells in confined spaces [91], involving the opening/closing of the gripping device. Microrobots that are magnetically actuated, such as Nelson's team system for eye surgery [92], have also offered some promise for minimally invasive surgical procedures. Magnetically actuated microtubes can be used to target diseases in other restricted areas of the human body. For instance, precise endovascular intervention can be carried out using submillimeter hydrogel-covered catheters with embedded hard magnetic particles using magnetic actuation [100]. Additionally, innovative and fascinating locomotion techniques, including rolling, walking, jumping, and crawling can be embedded into microrobots [55]. For example, Sitti's team [101] developed a device capable of multimodal mobility using dynamic magnetic fields. Recently, ultrasounds have been used to actuate micro- and nanorobots with exceptional tissue penetrating capabilities to perform surgical procedures at the cellular level [89, 90]. In addition to surgical applications, micro- and nanorobots have demonstrated great potential in biosensing tasks that aim to accurately diagnose diseases or even transport medications to specific cells to perform treatment [89]. All the exciting technological advances reported above have highlighted the great potential of micro- and nanorobots for performing precision clinical tasks at the cellular or even subcellular level. However, the ability of such tiny robots to address healthcare issues is in its infancy. Looking to the future, engineers, material scientists, and clinicians will have to cooperate to address current challenges and exploit the full potential of micro- and nanorobots in the medical field. The main challenges include (1) robot actuation and energy source for micromotors (engineering), (2) biocompatibility and surface properties (materials science, microfabrication), (3) interaction and cooperation between multiple micro- and nanorobots (swarm robotics), and (4) navigation (imaging and sensing). Finally, although micro- and nanorobots have shown promising results, their potential advantage over the state of the art (e.g., increased therapeutic efficacy, reduced patient discomfort and side effects, costs/benefit, etc.) must be proven to translate the technology from the lab to the operating room. Addressing these challenges will lead to accelerated translation of micro- and nanorobots technologies into practical clinical use, with potentially novel and more effective surgical and diagnostic workflows, which could lead to improving patients' life.

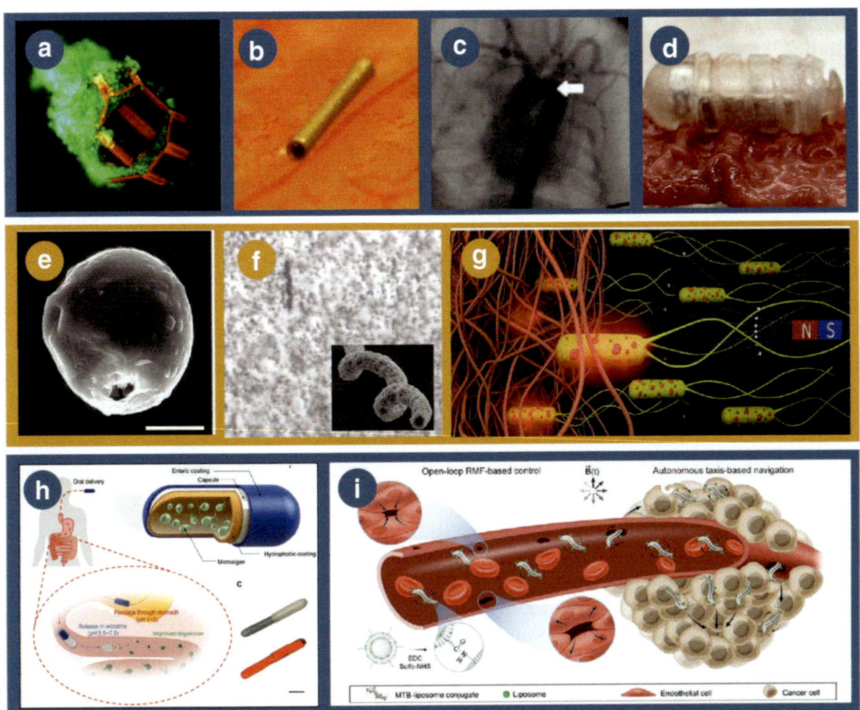

Fig. 3.5 Emerging micro-nano robots for surgical applications and drug delivery. (**a**) Untethered microgrippers capturing a cell (adapted from [91]); (**b**) tubular magnetic microrobot for eye surgery (adapted with John Wiley and Sons permission from [92]); (**c**) endovascular microrobot (adapted from [93] (CC BY 3.0)); (**d**) RoboCap, an orally ingestible robotic drug delivery capsule that locally clears the mucus layer, enhances luminal mixing, and topically deposits the drug payload in the small intestine to enhance drug absorption (adapted with AAAS permission from [94]); (**e**) scanning electron microscopy image of an ingestible micromotor that can navigate in the intestines enabling drug delivery applications (adapted with AAAS permission from [95]); (**f**) magnetic helical microrobot that can be remotely controlled to propel in complex biological fluids with high precision by using magnetic fields for image-guided targeted therapies (adapted with AAAS permission from [96]); (**g**) conceptual schematics of magnetically guided bacterial biohybrid microrobots for targeted localization and multistimuli-responsive drug release into tumours (adapted from [97] (CC BY 4.0)); (**h**) magnetic torque-driven microrobot can transport drugs inside a tumor via the vasculature (adapted with AAAS permission from [98]); (**i**) algae micromotors loaded within a swallowable capsule can deliver drugs in the gastrointestinal system (adapted with AAAS permission from [99])

3.5 Conclusions

In this chapter, we have provided an overview of the evolution of robotic surgery over the last few decades, which today has become a major area of innovation. At the infancy of robotic surgery, bulky industrial robots were used to perform clinical tasks. Since then, bespoke robotic surgical platforms have been designed specifically to be integrated into the surgical workflow. Surgical robots have become smaller, smarter, clinically usable, and well accepted by clinicians. Surgical robotics is interdisciplinary and involves the integration of imaging, sensing, computer vision, simulation, and human–machine interfaces. As such, it requires the cooperation and collaboration of experts from different fields, including engineering, medicine, computer science, materials science, and many others. While the technology is mature enough for many surgical applications, further technological advances are required toward the miniaturization and increased autonomy of surgical robots. In the future, with AI-driven miniaturized surgical robots, surgeries will become more patient specific and diagnosis and treatment at the same time (one-stop-shop) will become a reality. To this end, collaborations between academia, industry, and regulatory bodies are essential to translate new technologies from the lab to the clinical practice in an efficient way with realistic social-economic impacts.

References

1. Bergeles C, Yang G-Z. From passive tool holders to microsurgeons: safer, smaller, smarter surgical robots. IEEE Trans Biomed Eng. 2013;61(5):1565–76.
2. Troccaz J, Dagnino G, Yang G-Z. Frontiers of medical robotics: from concept to systems to clinical translation. Annu Rev Biomed Eng. 2019;21:193–218.
3. Troccaz J, Berkelman P, Cinquin P, et al. Interactive robots for medical applications. In: Lemke HU, Inamura K, Doi K, Vannier MW, Farman AG, Reiber JHC, editors. CARS 2002 computer assisted radiology and surgery. Berlin: Springer; 2002. p. 175–80.
4. Yang G-Z, Cambias J, Cleary K, et al. Medical robotics—regulatory, ethical, and legal considerations for increasing levels of autonomy. Am Assoc Adv Sci. 2017;2:eaam8638.
5. Vitiello V, Lee S-L, Cundy TP, et al. Emerging robotic platforms for minimally invasive surgery. IEEE Rev Biomed Eng. 2012;6:111–26.
6. Li QH, Zamorano L, Pandya A, et al. The application accuracy of the NeuroMate robot—a quantitative comparison with frameless and frame-based surgical localization systems. Comput Aided Surg. 2002;7(2):90–8.
7. Paul HA, Bargar WL, Mittlestadt B, et al. Development of a surgical robot for cementless total hip arthroplasty. Clin Orthop Relat Res. 1992;285:57–66.
8. Jakopec MY, Baena FR, Harris SJ, et al. The hands-on orthopaedic robot "Acrobot": early clinical trials of total knee replacement surgery. IEEE Trans Robot Autom. 2003;19(5):902–11.
9. Herry Y, Batailler C, Lording T, et al. Improved joint-line restitution in unicompartmental knee arthroplasty using a robotic-assisted surgical technique. Int Orthop. 2017;41(11):2265–71.
10. Lang J, Mannava S, Floyd A, et al. Robotic systems in orthopaedic surgery. J Bone Joint Surg. 2011;93(10):1296–9.
11. Marcus HJ, Cundy TP, Nandi D, et al. Robot-assisted and fluoroscopy-guided pedicle screw placement: a systematic review. Eur Spine J. 2014;23(2):291–7.
12. Schweikard A, Shiomi H, Adler J. Respiration tracking in radiosurgery without fiducials. Int J Med Robot Comput Assist Surg. 2005;1(2):19–27.
13. Butner SE, Ghodoussi M. Transforming a surgical robot for human telesurgery. IEEE Trans Robot Autom. 2003;19(5):818–24.
14. Guthart GS, Salisbury J K. The Intuitive/sup TM/telesurgery system: overview and application. In: Proceedings of the 2000 ICRA millennium conference IEEE international conference on robotics and automation symposia proceedings (Cat No 00CH37065). IEEE; 2000.
15. Feng Y, Guo Z, Dong Z, et al. An efficient cardiac mapping strategy for radiofrequency catheter ablation with active learning. Int J Comput Assist Radiol Surg. 2017;12(7):1199–207.

16. Rafii-Tari H, Payne CJ, Yang G-Z. Current and emerging robot-assisted endovascular catheterization technologies: a review. Ann Biomed Eng. 2014;42(4):697–715.
17. Mahmud E, Schmid F, Kalmar P, et al. Robotic peripheral vascular intervention with drug-coated balloons is feasible and reduces operator radiation exposure: results of the Robotic-Assisted Peripheral Intervention for Peripheral Artery Disease (RAPID) study II. J Invasive Cardiol. 2020;32(10):380–4.
18. Iwamoto SK, Tsai WS. Novel approaches utilizing robotic navigational bronchoscopy: a single institution experience. J Robot Surg. 2022;17:1001–6.
19. Valdastri P, Simi M, Webster RJ III. Advanced technologies for gastrointestinal endoscopy. Annu Rev Biomed Eng. 2012;14:397–429.
20. Beasley RA. Medical robots: current systems and research directions. J Robot. 2012;2012:401613.
21. Smith JA, Jivraj J, Wong R, et al. 30 years of neurosurgical robots: review and trends for manipulators and associated navigational systems. Ann Biomed Eng. 2016;44(4):836–46.
22. Howe RD, Matsuoka Y. Robotics for surgery. Annu Rev Biomed Eng. 1999;1(1):211–40.
23. Dogangil G, Davies B, Rodriguez Y, Baena F. A review of medical robotics for minimally invasive soft tissue surgery. Proc Inst Mech Eng H J Eng Med. 2010;224(5):653–79.
24. Davies B. A review of robotics in surgery. Proc Inst Mech Eng H J Eng Med. 2000;214(1):129–40.
25. Taylor RH, Menciassi A, Fichtinger G, et al. Medical robotics and computer-integrated surgery. In: Springer handbook of robotics. Berlin: Springer; 2016. p. 1657–84.
26. Camarillo DB, Krummel TM, Salisbury JK Jr. Robotic technology in surgery: past, present, and future. Am J Surg. 2004;188(4):2–15.
27. Rebello KJ. Applications of MEMS in surgery. Proc IEEE. 2004;92(1):43–55.
28. Menciassi A, Quirini M, Dario P. Microrobotics for future gastrointestinal endoscopy. Minim Invasive Ther Allied Technol. 2007;16(2):91–100.
29. Nelson BJ, Kaliakatsos IK, Abbott JJ. Microrobots for minimally invasive medicine. Annu Rev Biomed Eng. 2010;12:55–85.
30. Ciuti G, Menciassi A, Dario P. Capsule endoscopy: from current achievements to open challenges. IEEE Rev Biomed Eng. 2011;4:59–72.
31. Gilbert HB, Rucker DC, Webster RJ III. Concentric tube robots: the state of the art and future directions. In: Inaba M, Corke P, editors. Robotics research. Springer; 2016. p. 253–69.
32. Karas CS, Chiocca EA. Neurosurgical robotics: a review of brain and spine applications. J Robot Surg. 2007;1(1):39–43.
33. Yang G-Z, Bergeles C, Vitiello V. Surgical robotics: the next 25 years: successes, challenges, and the road ahead. UK-RAS Network; 2016.
34. Lee S-L, Lerotic M, Vitiello V, et al. From medical images to minimally invasive intervention: computer assistance for robotic surgery. Comput Med Imaging Graph. 2010;34(1):33–45.
35. Cundy TP, Shetty K, Clark J, et al. The first decade of robotic surgery in children. J Pediatr Surg. 2013;48(4):858–65.
36. Karimyan V, Sodergren M, Clark J, et al. Navigation systems and platforms in natural orifice translumenal endoscopic surgery. Int J Surg. 2009;7(4):297–304.
37. Marcus HJ, Hughes-Hallett A, Payne CJ, et al. Trends in the diffusion of robotic surgery: a retrospective observational study. Int J Med Robot Comput Assist Surg. 2017;13(4):e1870.
38. Kwoh YS, Hou J, Jonckheere EA, et al. A robot with improved absolute positioning accuracy for CT guided stereotactic brain surgery. IEEE Trans Biomed Eng. 1988;35(2):153–60.
39. Lavallee S, Troccaz J, Gaborit L, et al. Image guided operating robot: a clinical application in stereotactic neurosurgery. In: Proceedings of the 1992 IEEE international conference on robotics and automation. IEEE Computer Society; 1992.
40. Sutherland GR, Wolfsberger S, Lama S, et al. The evolution of neuroArm. Neurosurgery. 2013;72(Suppl_1):A27–32.
41. Cossetto T, Zareinia K, Sutherland G. Robotics for neurosurgery. In: Gomes P, editor. Medical robotics. Oxford: Elsevier; 2012. p. 59–77.

42. Chinzei K, Miller K. Towards MRI guided surgical manipulator. Med Sci Monit. 2001;7(1):153–63.
43. Joskowicz L, Shamir R, Freiman M, et al. Image-guided system with miniature robot for precise positioning and targeting in keyhole neurosurgery. Comput Aided Surg. 2006;11(4):181–93.
44. Hu X, Ohnmeiss DD, Lieberman IH. Robotic-assisted pedicle screw placement: lessons learned from the first 102 patients. Eur Spine J. 2013;22(3):661–6.
45. Bertelsen A, Melo J, Sánchez E, et al. A review of surgical robots for spinal interventions. Int J Med Robot Comput Assist Surg. 2013;9(4):407–22.
46. Paul HA, Mittlestadt B, Bargar WL, et al. A surgical robot for total hip replacement surgery. In: Proceedings of the ICRA. 1992.
47. Troccaz J, Peshkin M, Davies B. Guiding systems for computer-assisted surgery: introducing synergistic devices and discussing the different approaches. Med Image Anal. 1998;2(2):101–19.
48. Rosenberg LB. Virtual fixtures: perceptual tools for telerobotic manipulation. In: Proceedings of the IEEE virtual reality annual international symposium. IEEE; 1993.
49. Buschbaum J, Fremd R, Pohlemann T, et al. Computer-assisted fracture reduction: a new approach for repositioning femoral fractures and planning reduction paths. Int J Comput Assist Radiol Surg. 2015;10(2):149–59.
50. Westphal R, Winkelbach S, Wahl F, et al. Robot-assisted long bone fracture reduction. Int J Robot Res. 2009;28(10):1259–78.
51. Dagnino G, Georgilas I, Morad S, et al. Image-guided surgical robotic system for percutaneous reduction of joint fractures. Ann Biomed Eng. 2017;45(11):2648–62.
52. Dagnino G, Georgilas I, Köhler P, et al. Image-based robotic system for enhanced minimally invasive intra-articular fracture surgeries. In: Proceedings of the 2016 IEEE international conference on robotics and automation (ICRA). IEEE; 2016.
53. Dagnino G, Georgilas I, Köhler P, et al. Navigation system for robot-assisted intra-articular lower-limb fracture surgery. Int J Comput Assist Radiol Surg. 2016;11(10):1831–43.
54. Georgilas I, Dagnino G, Tarassoli P, et al. Robot-assisted fracture surgery: surgical requirements and system design. Ann Biomed Eng. 2018;46(10):1637–49.
55. Dupont PE, Nelson BJ, Goldfarb M, et al. A decade retrospective of medical robotics research from 2010 to 2020. Sci Robot. 2021;6(60):eabi8017.
56. Kraft B, Jäger C, Kraft K, et al. The AESOP robot system in laparoscopic surgery: increased risk or advantage for surgeon and patient? Surg Endosc Other Interv Tech. 2004;18(8):1216–23.
57. Ng W, Davies B, Hibberd R, et al. A first hand experience in transurethral resection of the prostate. IEEE Med Bio Soc Mag. 1993;12:120–5.
58. Marescaux J, Leroy J, Gagner M, et al. Transatlantic robot-assisted telesurgery. Nature. 2001;413(6854):379–80.
59. Bruns TL, Remirez AA, Emerson MA, et al. A modular, multi-arm concentric tube robot system with application to transnasal surgery for orbital tumors. Int J Robot Res. 2021;40(2–3):521–33.
60. Shang J, Leibrandt K, Giataganas P, et al. A single-port robotic system for transanal microsurgery—design and validation. IEEE Robot Automat Lett. 2017;2(3):1510–7.
61. Dagnino G, Kundrat D, Kwok TM, et al. In-vivo validation of a novel robotic platform for endovascular intervention. IEEE Trans Biomed Eng. 2023;70(6):1786–94.
62. Fagogenis G, Mencattelli M, Machaidze Z, et al. Autonomous robotic intracardiac catheter navigation using haptic vision. Sci Robot. 2019;4(29):eaaw1977.
63. Shang J, Noonan DP, Payne C, et al. An articulated universal joint based flexible access robot for minimally invasive surgery. In: Proceedings of the 2011 IEEE international conference on robotics and automation. IEEE; 2011.
64. Lee S, Constantinescu M, Chi W, et al. Devices for endovascular interventions: technical advances and translational challenges. NIHR white paper. 2017.
65. Kundrat D, Dagnino G, Kwok TM, et al. An MR-safe endovascular robotic platform: design, control, and ex-vivo evaluation. IEEE Trans Biomed Eng. 2021;68(10):3110–21.

66. Abdelaziz ME, Kundrat D, Pupillo M, et al. Toward a versatile robotic platform for fluoroscopy and MRI-guided endovascular interventions: a pre-clinical study. In: Proceedings of the 2019 IEEE/RSJ international conference on intelligent robots and systems (IROS). IEEE; 2019.
67. Dagnino G, Liu J, Abdelaziz ME, et al. Haptic feedback and dynamic active constraints for robot-assisted endovascular catheterization. In: Proceedings of the 2018 IEEE/RSJ international conference on intelligent robots and systems (IROS). IEEE; 2018.
68. Sears P, Dupont P. A steerable needle technology using curved concentric tubes. In: Proceedings of the 2006 IEEE/RSJ international conference on intelligent robots and systems. IEEE; 2006.
69. Webster RJ III. Design and mechanics of continuum robots for surgery. Baltimore: Johns Hopkins University; 2008.
70. Furusho J, Ono T, Murai R, et al. Development of a curved multi-tube (CMT) catheter for percutaneous umbilical blood sampling and control methods of CMT catheters for solid organs. In: Proceedings of the IEEE international conference mechatronics and automation, 2005. IEEE; 2005.
71. Gorini S, Quirini M, Menciassi A, et al. A novel SMA-based actuator for a legged endoscopic capsule. In: Proceedings of the the first IEEE/RAS-EMBS international conference on biomedical robotics and biomechatronics, 2006 BioRob 2006. IEEE; 2006.
72. Kwon J, Park S, Park J, et al. Evaluation of the critical stroke of an earthworm-like robot for capsule endoscopes. Proc Inst Mech Eng H J Eng Med. 2007;221(4):397–405.
73. Ciuti G, Valdastri P, Menciassi A, et al. Robotic magnetic steering and locomotion of capsule endoscope for diagnostic and surgical endoluminal procedures. Robotica. 2010;28(2):199–207.
74. Popek KM, Hermans T, Abbott JJ. First demonstration of simultaneous localization and propulsion of a magnetic capsule in a lumen using a single rotating magnet. In: Proceedings of the 2017 IEEE international conference on robotics and automation (ICRA). IEEE; 2017.
75. Simi M, Gerboni G, Menciassi A, et al. Magnetic mechanism for wireless capsule biopsy. J Med Devices. 2012;6(1):017611.
76. Kong K-C, Cha J, Jeon D, et al. A rotational micro biopsy device for the capsule endoscope. In: Proceedings of the 2005 IEEE/RSJ international conference on intelligent robots and systems. IEEE; 2005.
77. Chi W, Dagnino G, Kwok TM, et al. Collaborative robot-assisted endovascular catheterization with generative adversarial imitation learning. In: Proceedings of the 2020 IEEE international conference on robotics and automation (ICRA). IEEE; 2020.
78. Attanasio A, Scaglioni B, de Momi E, et al. Autonomy in surgical robotics. Annu Rev Control Robot Auton Syst. 2021;4:651–79.
79. Saeidi H, Opfermann J, Kam M, et al. Autonomous robotic laparoscopic surgery for intestinal anastomosis. Sci Robot. 2022;7(62):eabj2908.
80. Sutherland GR, Latour I, Greer AD, et al. An image-guided magnetic resonance-compatible surgical robot. Neurosurgery. 2008;62(2):286–93.
81. Groenhuis V, Siepel FJ, Stramigioli S. Sunram 5: a magnetic resonance-safe robotic system for breast biopsy, driven by pneumatic stepper motors. In: Nasab MHA, editor. Handbook of robotic and image-guided surgery. Oxford: Elsevier; 2020. p. 375–96.
82. Dagnino G, Georgilas I, Morad S, et al. Intra-operative fiducial-based CT/fluoroscope image registration framework for image-guided robot-assisted joint fracture surgery. Int J Comput Assist Radiol Surg. 2017;12(8):1383–97.
83. Dagnino G, Georgilas I, Tarassoli P, et al. Intra-operative 3D imaging system for robot-assisted fracture manipulation. In: Proceedings of the 2015 37th annual international conference of the IEEE Engineering in Medicine and Biology Society (EMBC). IEEE; 2015.
84. Markelj P, Tomaževič D, Likar B, et al. A review of 3D/2D registration methods for image-guided interventions. Med Image Anal. 2012;16(3):642–61.
85. Zhou X-Y, Lin J, Riga C, et al. Real-time 3-D shape instantiation from single fluoroscopy projection for fenestrated stent graft deployment. IEEE Robot Automat Lett. 2018;3(2):1314–21.

86. Pérez-Pachón L, Poyade M, Lowe T, et al. Image overlay surgery based on augmented reality: a systematic review. Adv Exp Med Biol. 2020;1260:175–95.
87. Glossop N. Localization and tracking technologies for medical robotics. In: Gomes P, editor. Medical robotics. Oxford: Elsevier; 2012. p. 41–58.
88. Chua Z, Jarc AM, Okamura AM. Toward force estimation in robot-assisted surgery using deep learning with vision and robot state. In: Proceedings of the 2021 IEEE international conference on robotics and automation (ICRA). IEEE; 2021.
89. Li J, de Ávila BE-F, Gao W, et al. Micro/nanorobots for biomedicine: delivery, surgery, sensing, and detoxification. Sci Robot. 2017;2(4):eaam6431.
90. Soto F, Chrostowski R. Frontiers of medical micro/nanorobotics: in vivo applications and commercialization perspectives toward clinical uses. Front Bioeng Biotechnol. 2018;6:170.
91. Leong TG, Randall CL, Benson BR, et al. Tetherless thermobiochemically actuated microgrippers. Proc Natl Acad Sci. 2009;106(3):703–8.
92. Chatzipirpiridis G, Ergeneman O, Pokki J, et al. Electroforming of implantable tubular magnetic microrobots for wireless ophthalmologic applications. Adv Healthc Mater. 2015;4(2):209–14.
93. Park S, Cha K, Park J. Development of biomedical microrobot for intravascular therapy. Int J Adv Robot Syst. 2010;7(1):1.
94. Srinivasan SS, Alshareef A, Hwang AV, et al. RoboCap: robotic mucus-clearing capsule for enhanced drug delivery in the gastrointestinal tract. Sci Robot. 2022;7(70):eabp9066.
95. Wu Z, Li L, Yang Y, et al. A microrobotic system guided by photoacoustic computed tomography for targeted navigation in intestines in vivo. Sci Robot. 2019;4(32):eaax0613.
96. Yan X, Zhou Q, Vincent M, et al. Multifunctional biohybrid magnetite microrobots for imaging-guided therapy. Sci Robot. 2017;2(12):eaaq1155.
97. Akolpoglu MB, Alapan Y, Dogan NO, et al. Magnetically steerable bacterial microrobots moving in 3D biological matrices for stimuli-responsive cargo delivery. Sci Adv. 2022;8(28):eabo6163.
98. Zhang F, Li Z, Duan Y, et al. Gastrointestinal tract drug delivery using algae motors embedded in a degradable capsule. Sci Robot. 2022;7(70):eabo4160.
99. Gwisai T, Mirkhani N, Christiansen MG, et al. Magnetic torque–driven living microrobots for increased tumor infiltration. Sci Robot. 2022;7(71):eabo0665.
100. Kim Y, Parada GA, Liu S, et al. Ferromagnetic soft continuum robots. Sci Robot. 2019;4(33):eaax7329.
101. Hu W, Lum GZ, Mastrangeli M, et al. Small-scale soft-bodied robot with multimodal locomotion. Nature. 2018;554(7690):81–5.

Therapeutic Training and Personal Assistance

4

Contents

4.1 Introduction

With an increasingly aged population all over the world and the prevalence of neurological and musculoskeletal disorders, the demand for rehabilitation and assistive devices is increasing. This chapter will provide a brief insight into the motivation for the development of rehabilitation and assistive robots. This chapter also emphasizes the clinical requirements and specific considerations for the development of these robots. For rehabilitation, available systems are mainly focused on recovering motor function of upper and lower limbs. In terms of robots for personal assistance, we categorize the current robotic systems into assistive robots for activities of daily living, mobile assistant robots, wearable exoskeletons for human augmentation, prosthetics, and social robots for cognitive assistance.

Y. Guo et al., *Medical Robotics*, Innovative Medical Devices,
https://doi.org/10.1007/978-981-99-7317-0_4

4.2 Motivations

The aging population is continuously increasing and has raised a series of healthcare challenges. According to the World Population Aging 2019 published by the United Nations, there are almost 703 million people aged 65 years or over, and this number is projected to double to 1.5 billion in 2050 [1]. As the elderly are susceptible to motor weakness, there is a great demand for personal assistance not only in hospitals but also in home-based environments [2].

In addition, for people with chronic diseases, cognitive or physical functions can be affected or continuously decline. Hence, therapeutic training is a critical way to help improve or recover these functions [3]. Furthermore, there are also many people with disabilities due to road accidents or major diseases. Intelligent prosthetics and mobile assistive robots can help amputees and disabled people to compensate with completing routine daily activities [4]. In this chapter, as illustrated in Fig. 4.1, we first take China as an example to analyze the potential social factors and then discuss the clinical demands that drive the development of rehabilitation and assistive robotics.

4.2.1 Social Factors: Taking China as an Example

4.2.1.1 Aging Population

China is the largest developing country and has the largest population in the world. According to the latest population census in 2021, there are over 1.4 billion people in China and around 18.70% of people are over 60 [5]. Consequently, there exist

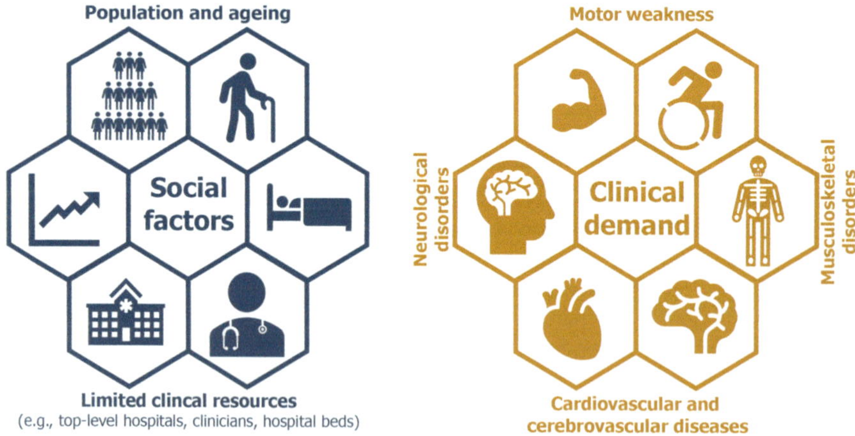

Fig. 4.1 Illustration of the social factors and clinical demands that drive the development of medical robotics. Rapid increase of the aging population and limited clinical resources (e.g., specialist hospitals and clinicians) are major social factors not only in China but all over the world. On the other hand, the prevalence of chronic diseases has raised significant requirements for clinical demand in disease management

major demands for healthcare and chronic disease management (e.g., stroke, dementia, etc.), particularly for age-related diseases [6]. Such a huge population of aging people will inevitably need sufficient and long-term medical resources not only in hospitals or rehabilitation centers but also in home-based environments [7].

4.2.1.2 Limited Clinical Resources

However, the reality is that there is a large gap between the demand and available medical resources, especially in rural areas. China has invested extensively in public health; however, there is a shortage of licensed doctors and registered nurses, with only 2.77 and 3.18 per 1000 people, respectively. This is well below the numbers of developed countries [8]. With only around 2749 AAA-level hospitals, there is a scarcity of high-quality medical resources in China, which is currently struggling to meet the medical needs of a large population. It's worth noting that this figure is even lower in other developing countries. There is also a major regional disparity between urban and rural areas and between developed and developing countries in terms of medical resource allocation [9]. Fullman et al. proposed a *Healthcare Access and Quality* (HAQ) index for measuring the medical resources of around 200 countries and territories [10], showing a highly correlated trend with the number of physicians, nurses, and hospital beds per thousand people. In their study, Iceland got the highest HAQ index, i.e., 97.1, whereas the values of some countries in Africa are lower than 25. The average HAQ index of China is 78, ranking 48th globally; however, the uneven distribution of medical resources leads to a large discrepancy between cities.

These social factors raise significant concerns for public health and medical resources. However, they also bring new opportunities for the development of new technologies for rehabilitation training and personal assistance. Hence, rehabilitation and assistive robotics have the potential to maintain a consistent standard of healthcare, while also alleviating the unequal distribution of medical resources and reducing the workload of medical personnel.

4.2.2 Clinical Demand

Research in human neuroscience has demonstrated that the prefrontal cortex, primary/secondary somatosensory cortex, primary motor cortex, supplementary motor area, and cingulate motor area are closely linked to human movement [11]. Apart from cortical areas, a number of subcortical regions, such as the cerebellum, basal ganglia, pontine nuclei, and thalamus, form networks that also have important roles in controlling human movement. The online commands of movement are first generated by the cortical regions related to motor functions, then transmitted to skeletal muscles through the spinal cord, and exhibited by the movement execution of limbs and body. Meanwhile, the sensory feedback acquired from different body parts is sent back to the somatosensory cortex, allowing the regulation of the movement. Furthermore, there is compelling evidence of brain connections linking the amygdala with the basal ganglia and the motor cortex, suggesting a two-way interaction between the networks responsible for movement and emotion [12].

Cognition is a complex psychological function that involves the mental process of obtaining knowledge and understanding through experience, thought, and the senses. It covers various aspects of intellectual functions and processes, such as perception, attention, thought, knowledge formation, memory and working memory, judgment and evaluation, reasoning and computation, problem-solving and decision-making, and language comprehension and production. People with impaired or degraded cognitive functions can encounter difficulties in daily life and social interaction, leading to an increased burden in caregiving.

Patients with musculoskeletal and neurological disorders require continuing medical attention. Motor weakness is common in the elderly. Additionally, the incidence rates of chronic disease, cardiovascular disease, musculoskeletal disease, and neurodegenerative disease are gradually rising, not only in the elderly population but also in younger groups [13–16].

The incidence, disability, and mortality rates of diseases are showing changing characteristics due to shifts in lifestyle and dietary habits [17]. Hence, the aforementioned issues mean a great demand for novel technologies to achieve high-quality, long-term, and personalized management of diseases [18, 19]. In this section, we mainly discuss major diseases that either affect a large population or bring a great burden to public health and medical resources. To manage these diseases, rehabilitation training can be performed routinely, which aims to either improve the patients with impaired/reduced motor or cognitive functions or maintain/delay the degradation of their functions. On the other hand, personal assistance focuses on compensating or augmenting human capability in daily activities, especially for people with missing functionalities.

4.2.2.1 Motor Weakness

With the increase of age, human beings can inevitably suffer from reduced motor function, originating from the relaxation of muscles, ligaments, and joints. Such weakness can lead to reduced stability and balance in movement, raising the risk of injury and falling. For example, elderly people with motor weakness will demonstrate reduced gait speed, step length, and range of motion during walking. Moreover, improper exercise can lead to sports injuries. Therefore, good exercise plans can help alleviate motor weakness. In addition, intelligent assistive devices are able to improve motor functions during daily life, as well as prevent falls.

4.2.2.2 Musculoskeletal Disorders

Osteoporosis and arthrophlogosis are common diseases of the musculoskeletal system. Patients with arthrophlogosis will suffer pain and stiffness of joints, especially after prolonged activities. It occurs in lower limbs, and patients can have abnormal gait patterns and pose difficulties in some postures, such as squatting and stooping [20]. Therefore, regular therapeutic training could slow down osteoporosis, and assistive robots may help with completing daily activities, preventing the aggravation of arthrophlogosis. Additionally, patients may exhibit similar impairment in motor functions after orthopedic. Rehabilitation training could accelerate the recovery of these patients. Nowadays, young people are increasingly keen to exercise;

however, the occurrence of sports injuries are also increasing. For people with severe injury, such as athletes, the appropriate rehabilitation training could speed up recovery and avoid undesired sequela.

4.2.2.3 Neurological Disorders

Dementia has become the leading neurological disease among the elderly, leading to impaired cognitive and physical functions, as shown in Fig. 4.2. The World Alzheimer Report 2021 [21] shows that there are over 55 million people worldwide living with dementia. This number is continually increasing and is projected to reach 78 million by 2030. Alzheimer's Disease (AD) is the most common form of dementia and has become the leading progressive neurodegenerative disease [22]. At present, it is estimated that 41 million cases of dementia, including AD, remain undiagnosed. AD is identified by a range of symptoms that include memory impairment, aphasia, apraxia, agnosia, impairment of visuospatial skills, executive dysfunction, and changes in personality and behavior. AD is most common in the elderly over 70 years old, leading to a significant burden on public health and caregivers [23].

Parkinson's Disease (PD) is the second most common neurological disorder that impacts human movement [24]. It affects 2–3% of individuals over the age of 65 [25]. The prevalence of PD increases with age, with aging being one of the leading causes. While rare in people under 40 years old, the average age of PD patients is approximately 60 years old. The loss of neurons that produce dopamine can result in a reduced amount of dopamine in the brain, which can lead to a decrease in the ability to control movement. This can manifest as slowing of movement and abnormalities in gait patterns [26]. Commonly, non-movement symptoms such as sleep disorders and visual deterioration, as well as movement difficulties like slow movement, tremors, rigidity, impaired posture, and gait, and cognitive issues such as depression and anxiety, are early symptoms experienced by patients with Parkinson's

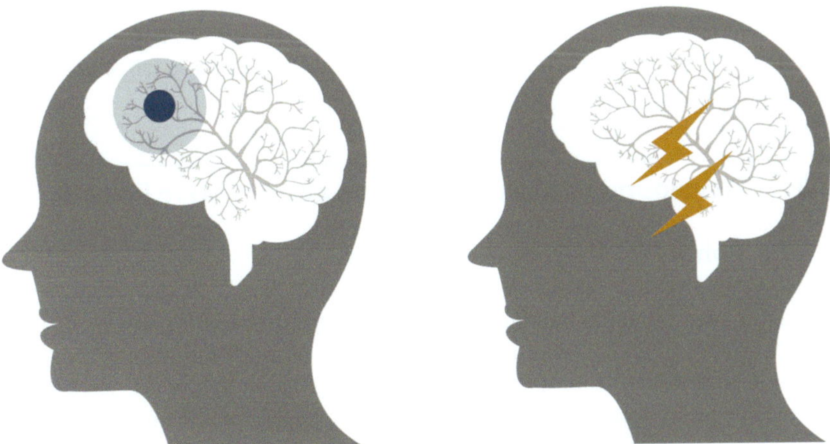

Fig. 4.2 Neurological disorders continuously affect human cognitive function

disease. For those at an advanced stage of the disease progression, the freezing of gait becomes more apparent, which significantly influences their quality of life.

Autism Spectrum Disorder (ASD) is a wide range of neurodevelopmental disorders, mainly manifested as speech disorders, social communication disorders, and emotional perception disorders [27]. ASD affects approximately 78 million people worldwide [28], and it has become a condition of global importance due to the effects on individuals and families. As tremendous heterogeneity exists among individuals with ASD, the development of universal clinical treatments for ASD is quite challenging. Currently, early diagnosis and intervention are the main methods for this disease [29, 30]. The fact is that the majority of autism patients do not have access to adequate healthcare, education, and social care services. Hence, the need for robot-assisted personalized intervention and social assistance in home-based environments is of paramount significance.

4.2.2.4 Cardiovascular Disease

Cardiovascular and cerebrovascular diseases, such as stroke, ischemic heart disease, and hypertensive heart disease, are the significant causes of death and disability worldwide. Stroke, in particular, ranked second as a cause of death and third as a cause of death and disability in 2019 [31]. The report indicated that in 2019 [31], there were 12.2 million new cases of stroke and a total of 101 million existing cases of stroke worldwide. Additionally, China has been identified as the country with the highest risk of stroke globally [16].

Patients who survive a stroke will manifest major degradation of musculoskeletal and/or neurological systems, especially on the affected side. Evidence has shown that stroke patients have a greater chance of restoring and recovering motor function after therapeutic training [3]. Therefore, it is crucial to offer patients who have suffered from a stroke with extended rehabilitation training. However, it is unfortunate that not all stroke patients have the opportunity to undergo rehabilitation therapy while in the hospital. For example, in China, only 30–60% of stroke patients receive rehabilitation therapy after their initial neurology or neurosurgery treatment. Furthermore, less than 10% of these patients are able to undergo any other forms of therapy [32]. Hence, these situations pose significant needs for rehabilitation and assistive robots.

4.3 Development of Rehabilitation and Assistive Robotics

4.3.1 Robots for Therapeutic Training

The aim of rehabilitation training is to improve the movement capability of patients with neurological and/or musculoskeletal disorders through multidisciplinary treatments. Compared to labor-intensive work performed by therapists, rehabilitation robots can automatically aid patients in practicing specific functional movements, as well as provide a quantitative assessment of the rehabilitation performance [33, 34]. There have been various rehabilitation training robots developed in the past decades, which can be categorized into two main categories: end-effector-based and exoskeleton-based [35, 36].

End-effector robots are designed to control the motion of the furthest part of limbs and are easy to set up. However, they may also cause unintended movement in other joints. In contrast, exoskeleton robots have complex mechanical designs to control the movement of joints and links. Moreover, exoskeletons are wearable robots that are well-suited to the anatomical axes of the human body. Rehabilitation for the upper extremities primarily aims to restore patients' ability to reach and grasp, while lower-limb rehabilitation usually involves standing, walking, and balance training. In order to keep patients engaged in their rehabilitation, robots are designed to detect human movement intentions and provide informative biofeedback through various HMIs while performing these exercises. Therapeutic robots, on the other hand, are desired to accurately evaluate the quality of movement by measuring several biosignals and kinematic and kinetic parameters from patients.

MIT-MANUS is one of the first rehabilitation training robots that achieved successful commercial applications during the past decades [37]. Through the use of a parallelogram linkage driven by three geared actuators, this robotic system is able to guide the movement of a subject's upper limb with 2-DoF elbow and forearm motion and 3-DoF wrist motion. In addition, impedance control was introduced to offer safe, stable, and compliant operation in close physical contact with humans. In 1999, MIME was developed by Stanford University, which utilized a Puma-560 robotic arm to guide the 3DoF motion of the affected side by reproducing the movement of the patient's health side [38].

During rehabilitation training, interaction games are widely incorporated into rehabilitation training robots, thus improving the engagement of patients. Along with various sensing techniques, such as joint velocity, torque, and *Electromyography* (EMG), the evaluation of patients' physical functions can be simultaneously performed. Recently, advanced *Virtual Reality* (VR) and *Augmented Reality* (AR) technologies have been combined into therapeutic robotic systems, which can enhance the engagement of users and guide them for training in a controlled environment during robot-assist training [39].

In addition to training for people with physical impairment, the use of rehabilitation training robots for assisting intervention for patients with cognitive impairment is urgent as the number of these patients (such as AD, PD, and ASD) is significantly increasing all over the world. Particularly, interactive games are specifically designed for memory exercises. They can assess an individual's short-term and spatial memory. These dysfunctions have been shown to be the main symptoms in patients with AD and dementia [40].

4.3.2 Robots for Personal Assistance

Assistive robots are designed to assist patients with physical impairments in performing their desired movements. This is achieved through continuous interactions between the patient and the robot, which can either augment or compensate for the patient's physical limitations in a robotic-assisted manner [18, 41]. As illustrated in Fig. 4.3, assistive robots can take on various forms depending on the specific practical needs of different users. These forms include exoskeletons, prostheses, mobile assistive robots, and social robots. Through the use of assistive robots, users can improve their quality of life by restoring or enhancing their functional movement in ADL.

4.3.2.1 Assistive Robots for ADL

For patients with impaired physical functions, there is a pressing need for developing assistance devices that are able to help them complete daily activities, such as eating, drinking, washing, and teeth cleaning. The first commercialized assistive robot for ADL, namely Handy1, was developed in 1987. Handy1 is a robotic system that is capable of assisting the most severely disabled with several ADL applications [42]. For instance, a number of robotic feeders were developed for dining assistance of individuals who lack upper extremity function. Such robots are typically mounted in a fixed place. Some advanced versions can help patients complete eating automatically by integrating with face and mouth recognition techniques.

4.3.2.2 Mobile Assistive Robots

For people with impaired function of lower limbs, assistive robots incorporated with mobile platforms (e.g., intelligent wheelchair or patient transfer robot)

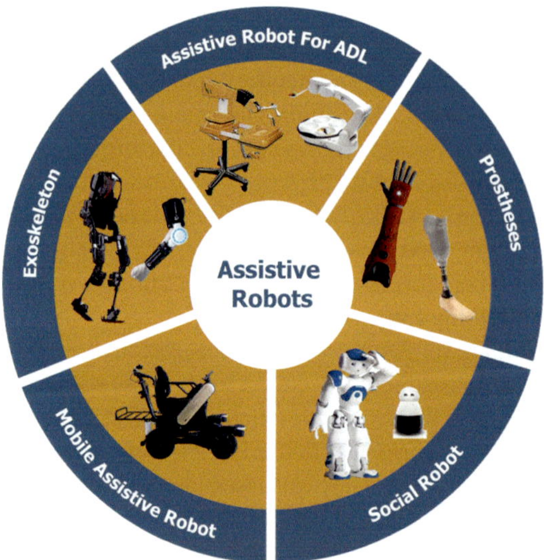

Fig. 4.3 Different types of assistive robots that can either restore or augment the functional movement in ADL, including assistive robots for ADL (Handy 1, adapted with Springer Nature permission from [42]; Obi, Obi, © 2023), exoskeletons (Rewalk, ReWalk Robotics, © 2023; HAL, copyright by CYBERDYNE Inc.), prostheses (C-Leg4, copyright by Ottobock; Hero Arm, Open Bionics, © 2022), mobile assistive robots (Whill, WHILL Inc., © 2015–2023), and social robots (NAO and Kuri, images are with CC BY 4.0 license)

enable the users to achieve free movement and automatic navigation in the free-living environment [43]. One of the main focuses during the development of these mobile assistive robots is to understand the environment around them (such as mapping and localization) and how they interact with it [44, 45]. Additionally, various mobile assistive robots integrated with robotic arms can provide the augmented capabilities of patients to complete complicated ADL [46], such as opening a door or grasping objects. Another group of mobile assistive robots is telepresence robots, which enable monitoring and simulate face-to-face interaction between the patient and their doctors or family members remotely [47]. Moreover, mobile assistive robots integrated with intelligent algorithms can help perform 24/7 hour healthcare monitoring at home, such as gait analysis and fall prevention [48].

4.3.2.3 Wearable Exoskeletons for Human Augmentation

Wearable exoskeletons consist of joints and links that are aligned with the anatomical axes of the human body. Upper-limb exoskeletons aim to guide the movement of the elbow and/or shoulder joints through the dedicated mechanical design to assist or resist the joint movement [49, 50]. Robotic exoskeletons for lower limbs usually have motorized joints at the hip, knee, and ankle. They are designed to enhance the walking and running abilities of patients with spinal cord injuries, stroke, or other conditions that affect their ability to walk [51, 52]. Robotic gloves can enhance patients' hand movements by controlling their fingers and wrists, promoting functional grasping in cases of pathologies [53, 54].

In 2000, the first version of Lokomat [55], a grounded exoskeleton for gait training, was developed by Hocoma (Hocoma, Volketswil, Switzerland). The Lokomat is a robotic treadmill training system, while a bodyweight support system is used to suspend individuals and their legs are attached to robotic legs. For wearable exoskeletons for the lower limb, the first clinical trial for the ReWalk was held at MossRehab located in Philadelphia in 2009. Soft wearable exoskeletons are quickly becoming more prevalent thanks to recent advancements in material sciences and robotics [56]. When compared to traditional rigid countermeasures, the compliant nature of soft robotics allows for safe interaction with humans and reduces restrictions on anatomical joint alignment [57]. Except for the development of exoskeletons for rehabilitation training, such wearable devices have been used to augment human power in some tedious tasks, such as running and lifting [58, 59].

4.3.2.4 Prostheses

Prostheses are artificial replacements that can restore motor functions related to missing body parts, which are able to assist amputees and paralyzed people to complete ADL independently. Moreover, extensive research effort has been applied to the development of active prostheses incorporating a bidirectional HMI [34]. Robotic prostheses offer the ability to detect a user's motion intention and execute the desired movements, while also providing sensory information as feedback. By utilizing advanced mechatronics, sensing, and control technologies, these prostheses can receive online commands from amputees, allowing for a more natural range of motion [60, 61]. The integration of these technologies results in a professional and effective solution for those in need of prosthetic limbs.

4.3.2.5 Social Robots for Cognition Assistance

Another line of research on assistive robotics is the development of social robotics, which is a relatively new field. It involves interdisciplinary research, including artificial intelligence, machine learning, psychology, medicine, social and cognitive sciences, neuroscience, and human–computer interaction [30, 62]. Specifically, social robotics can be defined as an autonomous robot that can follow social behaviors and norms conforming to its own identity, capture rich and dynamic social activities and environmental information of human targets, and interact and communicate with humans in daily living environments [62].

With the rapid development of sensors, computer vision, artificial intelligence, microelectronics, and other related technologies, social robots integrated with multimodal sensing have been widely used in different social and health fields in recent years, including entertainment, early childhood education, elderly, autistic children, and neurodegenerative intervention applications [29, 63–65]. Taking autism as an example, social robots that are able to provide intervention and treatment can be widely deployed in hospital and home-based environments. They can not only provide long-term monitoring or rehabilitation for emotion, perception, and memory disorders but also help explore brain development and the inherent law of processing information by using longitudinal data, thus enabling personalized intervention and rehabilitation strategies [29, 65].

4.4 Conclusions

Aging and limited medical resources are major social factors that drive the development of rehabilitation and assistive robots. Musculoskeletal and neurological disorders have become prevalent in modern society, leading to many patients suffering from degraded physical and cognitive functions. In addition, most patients who survive stroke have impaired motor functions. For amputees or paralyzed people, lost functions need to be restored in order to maintain physical function and dignity. Hence, the development of rehabilitation and assistive robotics has become important in medical robotics.

Although we have witnessed successful applications of many rehabilitation and assistive robots in recent decades, personal requirements for rehabilitation and assistive robots are highly diverse and patient specific. It should also be emphasized that rehabilitation and assistive robots work closely with human users in daily life, for which safety and intelligent HRI are of significant importance in system design and control. It is believed that in the near future robotic systems will be more lightweight, comfortable, and intelligent, providing personalized and effective treatment and assistance.

References

1. World population ageing 2019. United Nations, Department of Economic and Social Affairs. 2019.
2. Christensen K, Doblhammer G, Rau R, et al. Ageing populations: the challenges ahead. Lancet. 2009;374(9696):1196–208.
3. Langhorne P, Bernhardt J, Kwakkel G. Stroke rehabilitation. Lancet. 2011;377(9778):1693–702.
4. Clegg A, Young J, Iliffe S, et al. Frailty in elderly people. Lancet. 2013;381(9868):752–62.
5. Wang X-Q, Chen P-J. Population ageing challenges health care in China. Lancet. 2014;383(9920):870.
6. Beard JR, Officer A, de Carvalho IA, et al. The World report on ageing and health: a policy framework for healthy ageing. Lancet. 2016;387(10033):2145–54.
7. Feng Z, Glinskaya E, Chen H, et al. Long-term care system for older adults in China: policy landscape, challenges, and future prospects. Lancet. 2020;396(10259):1362–72.
8. Statistical Communique of People's Republic of China on the 2019 Health. National Health Commission of People's Republic of China; 2020.
9. Chai K-C, Zhang Y-B, Chang K-C. Regional disparity of medical resources and its effect on mortality rates in China. Front Public Health. 2020;8:8.
10. Fullman N, Yearwood J, Abay SM, et al. Measuring performance on the Healthcare Access and Quality Index for 195 countries and territories and selected subnational locations: a systematic analysis from the Global Burden of Disease Study 2016. Lancet. 2018;391(10136):2236–71.
11. Grafton ST, Hamilton AFDC. Evidence for a distributed hierarchy of action representation in the brain. Hum Mov Sci. 2007;26(4):590–616.
12. Koziol LF, Budding D, Andreasen N, et al. Consensus paper: the cerebellum's role in movement and cognition. Cerebellum. 2014;13(1):151–77.
13. Clark NM. Management of chronic disease by patients. Annu Rev Public Health. 2003;24(1):289–313.
14. Brooks PM. The burden of musculoskeletal disease—a global perspective. Clin Rheumatol. 2006;25(6):778–81.
15. Hou Y, Dan X, Babbar M, et al. Ageing as a risk factor for neurodegenerative disease. Nat Rev Neurol. 2019;15(10):565–81.
16. Johnson CO, Nguyen M, Roth GA, et al. Global, regional, and national burden of stroke, 1990–2016: a systematic analysis for the Global Burden of Disease Study 2016. Lancet Neurol. 2019;18(5):439–58.
17. Afshin A, Sur PJ, Fay KA, et al. Health effects of dietary risks in 195 countries, 1990–2017: a systematic analysis for the Global Burden of Disease Study 2017. Lancet. 2019;393(10184):1958–72.
18. Chase A. New assistive devices for stroke rehabilitation. Nat Rev Neurol. 2014;10(2):59.
19. Broekens J, Heerink M, Rosendal H. Assistive social robots in elderly care: a review. Geron. 2009;8(2):94–103.
20. Hsu W-L, Chen C-Y, Tsauo J-Y, et al. Balance control in elderly people with osteoporosis. J Formos Med Assoc. 2014;113(6):334–9.
21. World Alzheimer report 2021. Alzheimer's Disease International; 2022.
22. Reitz C, Mayeux R. Alzheimer disease: epidemiology, diagnostic criteria, risk factors and biomarkers. Biochem Pharmacol. 2014;88(4):640–51.
23. Mohamed S, Rosenheck R, Lyketsos CG, et al. Caregiver burden in Alzheimer disease: cross-sectional and longitudinal patient correlates. Am J Geriatr Psychiatry. 2010;18(10):917–27.
24. Poewe W, Seppi K, Tanner CM, et al. Parkinson disease. Nat Rev Dis Primers. 2017;3(1):1–21.
25. Dorsey E, Sherer T, Okun MS, et al. The emerging evidence of the Parkinson pandemic. J Parkinsons Dis. 2018;8(s1):S3–8.
26. Armstrong MJ, Okun MS. Diagnosis and treatment of Parkinson disease: a review. JAMA. 2020;323(6):548–60.

27. Johnson CP, Myers SM. Identification and evaluation of children with autism spectrum disorders. Pediatrics. 2007;120(5):1183–215.
28. Lord C, Charman T, Havdahl A, et al. The Lancet Commission on the future of care and clinical research in autism. Lancet. 2022;399(10321):271–334.
29. Scassellati B, Boccanfuso L, Huang C-M, et al. Improving social skills in children with ASD using a long-term, in-home social robot. Sci Robot. 2018;3(21):eaat7544.
30. Yang G-Z, Dario P, Kragic D. Social robotics—trust, learning, and social interaction. Am Assoc Adv Sci. 2018;3:eaau8839.
31. Feigin VL, Stark BA, Johnson CO, et al. Global, regional, and national burden of stroke and its risk factors, 1990–2019: a systematic analysis for the Global Burden of Disease Study 2019. Lancet Neurol. 2021;20(10):795–820.
32. Wu S, Wu B, Liu M, et al. Stroke in China: advances and challenges in epidemiology, prevention, and management. Lancet Neurol. 2019;18(4):394–405.
33. Tejima N. Rehabilitation robotics: a review. Adv Robot. 2001;14(7):551–64.
34. Guo Y, Gu X, Yang G-Z. Human–robot interaction for rehabilitation robotics. In: Glauner P, Plugmann P, Lerzynski G, editors. Digitalization in healthcare. Cham: Springer; 2021. p. 269–95.
35. Chang WH, Kim YH. Robot-assisted therapy in stroke rehabilitation. J Stroke. 2013;15(3):174–81.
36. Molteni F, Gasperini G, Cannaviello G, et al. Exoskeleton and end-effector robots for upper and lower limbs rehabilitation: narrative review. PM&R. 2018;10(9):S174–S88.
37. Krebs HI, Hogan N, Aisen ML, et al. Robot-aided neurorehabilitation. IEEE Trans Rehabil Eng. 1998;6(1):75–87.
38. Lum PS, Burgar CG, van der Loos M, et al. MIME robotic device for upper-limb neurorehabilitation in subacute stroke subjects: a follow-up study. J Rehabil Res Dev. 2006;43(5):631.
39. Mubin O, Alnajjar F, Jishtu N, et al. Exoskeletons with virtual reality, augmented reality, and gamification for stroke patients' rehabilitation: systematic review. JMIR Rehabil Assist Technol. 2019;6(2):e12010.
40. Vovk A, Patel A, Chan D. Augmented reality for early Alzheimer's disease diagnosis. In: Proceedings of the extended abstracts of the 2019 CHI conference on human factors in computing systems. 2019.
41. Brose SW, Weber DJ, Salatin BA, et al. The role of assistive robotics in the lives of persons with disability. Am J Phys Med Rehabil. 2010;89(6):509–21.
42. Topping M. An overview of the development of handy 1, a rehabilitation robot to assist the severely disabled. J Intell Robot Syst. 2002;34:253–63.
43. Montesano L, Díaz M, Bhaskar S, et al. Towards an intelligent wheelchair system for users with cerebral palsy. IEEE Trans Neural Syst Rehabil Eng. 2010;18(2):193–202.
44. Mur-Artal R, Tardós JD. ORB-SLAM2: an open-source slam system for monocular, stereo, and RGB-D cameras. IEEE Trans Robot. 2017;33(5):1255–62.
45. Hess W, Kohler D, Rapp H, et al. Real-time loop closure in 2D LIDAR SLAM. In: Proceedings of the 2016 IEEE international conference on robotics and automation (ICRA). IEEE; 2016.
46. Ktistakis IP, Bourbakis NG. Assistive intelligent robotic wheelchairs. IEEE Potent. 2017;36(1):10–3.
47. Moyle W, Jones C, Cooke M, et al. Connecting the person with dementia and family: a feasibility study of a telepresence robot. BMC Geriatr. 2014;14(1):1–11.
48. Guo Y, Deligianni F, Gu X, et al. 3-D canonical pose estimation and abnormal gait recognition with a single RGB-D camera. IEEE Robot Automat Lett. 2019;4(4):3617–24.
49. Lo HS, Xie SQ. Exoskeleton robots for upper-limb rehabilitation: state of the art and future prospects. Med Eng Phys. 2012;34(3):261–8.
50. Samper-Escudero JL, Giménez-Fernandez A, Sánchez-Urán MÁ, et al. A cable-driven exosuit for upper limb flexion based on fibres compliance. IEEE Access. 2020;8:153297–310.
51. Liu W, Yin B, Yan B. A survey on the exoskeleton rehabilitation robot for the lower limbs. In: Proceedings of the 2016 2nd international conference on control, automation and robotics (ICCAR). IEEE; 2016.

52. Rodríguez-Fernández A, Lobo-Prat J, Font-Llagunes JM. Systematic review on wearable lower-limb exoskeletons for gait training in neuromuscular impairments. J Neuroeng Rehabil. 2021;18(1):1–21.
53. Polygerinos P, Wang Z, Galloway KC, et al. Soft robotic glove for combined assistance and at-home rehabilitation. Robot Auton Syst. 2015;73:135–43.
54. Cheng N, Phua KS, Lai HS, et al. Brain-computer interface-based soft robotic glove rehabilitation for stroke. IEEE Trans Biomed Eng. 2020;67(12):3339–51.
55. Jezernik S, Colombo G, Keller T, et al. Robotic orthosis lokomat: a rehabilitation and research tool. Neuromodulation. 2003;6(2):108–15.
56. Rus D, Tolley MT. Design, fabrication and control of soft robots. Nature. 2015;521(7553):467–75.
57. Walsh C. Human-in-the-loop development of soft wearable robots. Nat Rev Mater. 2018;3(6):78–80.
58. Ding Y, Kim M, Kuindersma S, et al. Human-in-the-loop optimization of hip assistance with a soft exosuit during walking. Sci Robot. 2018;3(15):eaar5438.
59. Yun S-S, Kim K, Ahn J, et al. Body-powered variable impedance: an approach to augmenting humans with a passive device by reshaping lifting posture. Sci Robot. 2021;6(57):eabe1243.
60. Musallam S, Corneil B, Greger B, et al. Cognitive control signals for neural prosthetics. Science. 2004;305(5681):258–62.
61. Mendez V, Iberite F, Shokur S, et al. Current solutions and future trends for robotic prosthetic hands. Annu Rev Control Robot Auton Syst. 2021;4:595–627.
62. Breazeal C, Dautenhahn K, Kanda T. Social robotics. In: Siciliano B, Khatib O, editors. Springer handbook of robotics. Cham: Springer; 2016. p. 1935–72.
63. Pennisi P, Tonacci A, Tartarisco G, et al. Autism and social robotics: a systematic review. Autism Res. 2016;9(2):165–83.
64. Góngora Alonso S, Hamrioui S, de la Torre Díez I, et al. Social robots for people with aging and dementia: a systematic review of literature. Telemed e-Health. 2019;25(7):533–40.
65. Jain S, Thiagarajan B, Shi Z, et al. Modeling engagement in long-term, in-home socially assistive robot interventions for children with autism spectrum disorders. Sci Robot. 2020;5(39):eaaz3791.

Rehabilitation and Assistive Robotics

5

Contents

5.1 Introduction

As introduced in Chap. 4, there exist diverse social factors and significant clinical demands that drive the development of rehabilitation and assistive robots. This chapter aims to provide an overview of the technical aspects of rehabilitation and assistive robotics. We will consider in sequence robots for therapeutic training, personal assistance, cognitive assistance, and prosthetics. For each category, key technological advantages and limitations are discussed. Since rehabilitation and assistive robots need to closely interact with human beings, we will emphasize the importance of HRI and different HMIs. This chapter also introduces emerging technologies in soft actuation, multimodal interfaces, and robot control strategies.

Y. Guo et al., *Medical Robotics*, Innovative Medical Devices,
https://doi.org/10.1007/978-981-99-7317-0_5

5.2 Robots for Therapeutic Training

In order to improve patients' physical functions, effective therapies are needed to help patients recover from stroke or other musculoskeletal/neurological disorders. Conventional therapeutic methods mainly depend on intensive and frequent intervention provided by professional therapists. Robots showing superiority in endurance and efficiency can automatically support patients in practicing specific functional movements as well as providing a quantitative assessment of the rehabilitation performance [1–3]. Figure 5.1 illustrates the development of robots for therapeutic training, starting from end-effector-based robots to grounded exoskeletons and then moving to wearable exoskeletons in recent years.

Conventional end-effector-based robots aim to guide the movement of the most distal segment of limbs (e.g., hand and foot) [4, 5]. These systems are either built upon industrial robotic arms or based on multiple linkage structures. The advantages of end-effector-based systems lie in several aspects, such as being simple in structure, easy to build and control, and low in cost. However, these systems can be cumbersome, and they do not consider the posture and position information of other joints of the upper limb, leading to motion compensation or potential trauma during training.

To overcome the inherent limitations of end-effector-based robotic systems, extensive research interest has been gained in exoskeletons [2, 6]. Exoskeletons are wearable robots that are placed on the user's limb, aiming to augment or restore human movement by guiding each joint individually. Made out of rigid or soft materials, they are composed of several motors or driving modules aligned with key

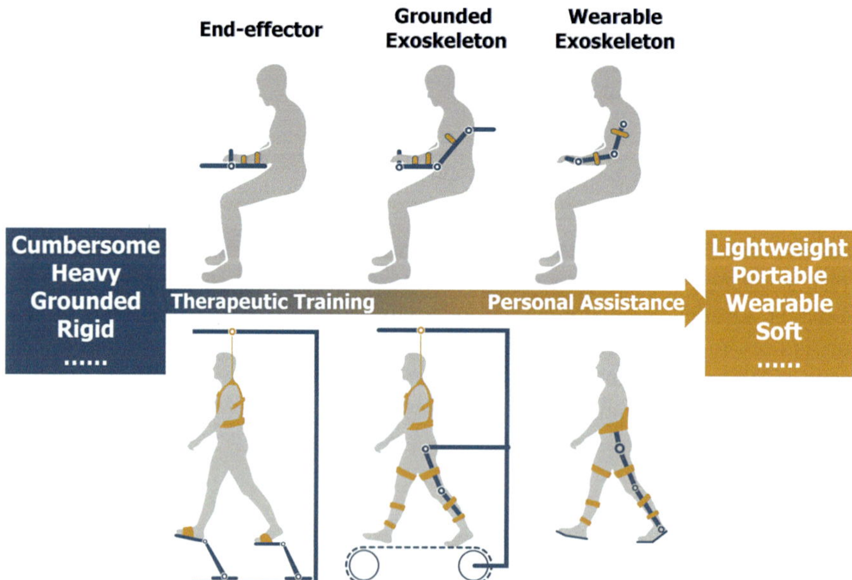

Fig. 5.1 Evolution of robotic systems for therapeutic training and personal assistance

body joints. Compared to end-effector-based robots, exoskeletons are capable of guiding the movement of each joint individually and providing a larger RoM, thus enabling rehabilitation with more flexibility. As illustrated in Fig. 5.1, early attempts were focused on grounded exoskeletons, where the entire system can be large and heavy, limiting the therapeutic training in equally limited scenarios. More recently, lightweight and wearable exoskeletons have gained increasing popularity, which can not only provide rehabilitation training anytime and anywhere but also enable personal assistance in daily life.

5.2.1 Upper-Limb Rehabilitation Robots

For human beings, most daily activities (e.g., grasping and manipulating objects) are accomplished using upper limbs. Hence, the rehabilitation of upper limbs is of paramount significance. However, the high DoFs of upper limbs raise challenges in developing therapeutic robots. An upper limb is composed of the shoulder, elbow, wrist joints, and fingers. For shoulder and wrist joints, there exist three DoFs each and one DoF for the elbow joint. A hand is more complex, with a total of 19 DoFs. In general, each kinematic joint can be viewed as a hinge; therefore, an upper limb can be modeled by the interconnections of multiple rigid bodies. Such a complex structure leads to a large RoM and diverse movements.

Early research focused on end-effector-based robots for upper limb rehabilitation. The mechanical design of end-effector-based robots intends to restrain human hand dexterity and then guide users to perform specific exercises. Commonly, interactive games are designed to offer specific rehabilitation protocols as well as to enhance the engagement of participants. Such a scheme also forms a closed-loop rehabilitation training for the patients from visual perception to motor control. MIT-MANUS, as shown in the first row of Fig. 5.2, was the first end-effector-based rehabilitation robot developed by MIT [4]. It has been successfully commercialized into Inmotion ARM (Bionik, Massachusetts, US). While training with MIT-MANUS, participants need to grasp/move the handle and watch the monitor to complete the interaction games. The advantages of end-effector-based systems lie in several aspects, such as being simple in structure, easy to build and control, and low in cost. However, these systems are cumbersome and do not consider the posture and position of other joints of the upper limb. Therefore, by training with the end-effector-based systems, patients may produce movements that the upper limb cannot achieve or have to use compensatory movements. Meanwhile, grasping the handle cannot guarantee desired movements, forces, and torques of the upper limb, which may lead to potential secondary trauma.

To overcome the inherent challenges of end-effector-based robotic systems, exoskeletons consisting of a series of structures connected to the upper limb have been extensively studied [12]. Compared to end-effector-based approaches, they are advantageous in providing assistance for each joint individually and supporting a large RoM for the upper limbs [5]. Early exoskeletons, as shown in the lower part of Fig. 5.2, are grounded systems. One of the representative grounded exoskeletons is

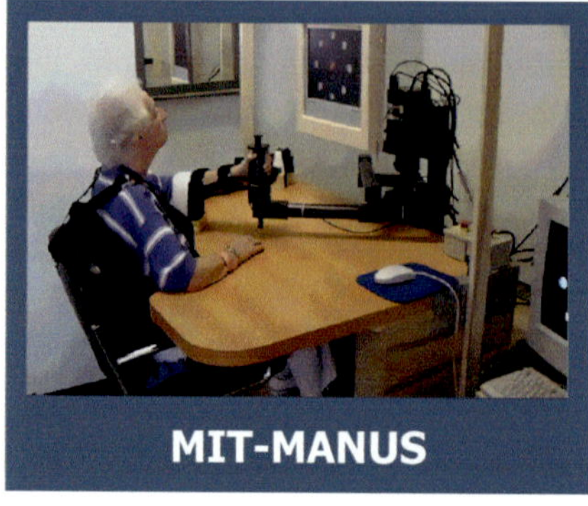

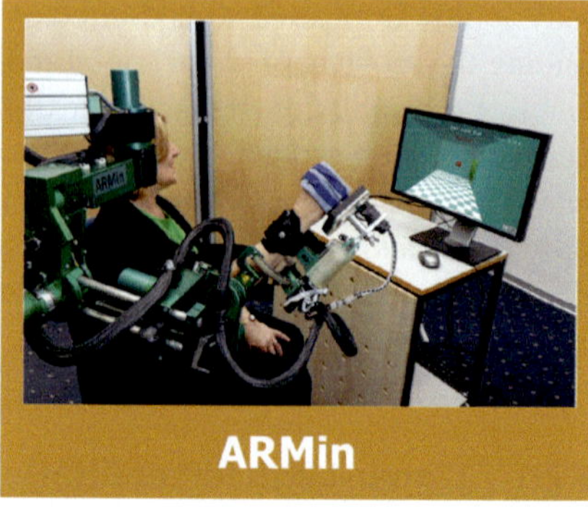

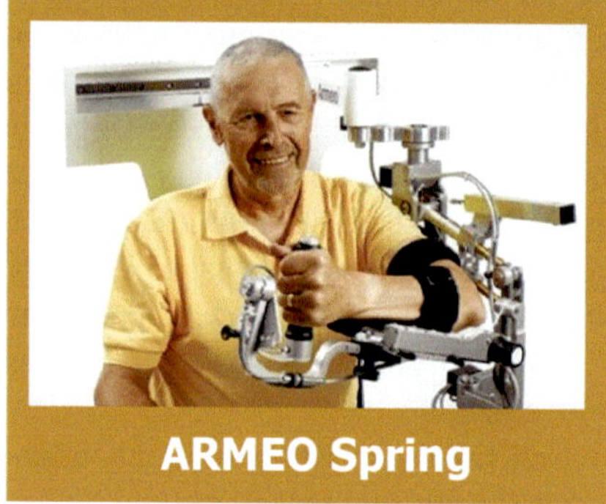

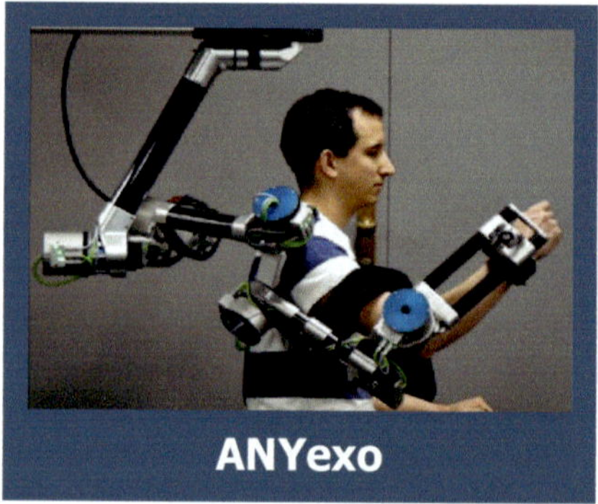

Fig. 5.2 Representative end-effector-based robots and grounded exoskeletons for upper limb rehabilitation and assistance. MIT-MANUS [4] (adapted with Taylor & Francis permission from [7]), commercialized as Inmotion ARM (Bionik, Massachusetts, US), ARMin [8] (adapted from [9] (CC BY 4.0)), AMERO Spring [10] (Hocoma, Volketswil, Switzerland; Hocoma, © 2023), and ANYexo (adapted with IEEE permission from [11])

ARMin developed by ETH [8], which consists of seven active DoFs and an arm length that can be manually adjusted according to patients' biometrics. Task-oriented interaction games were integrated with the ARMin system, enhancing the engagement of users and facilitating rehabilitation. However, grounded exoskeletons can be large and heavy, requiring patients to sit in a fixed place to complete therapeutic training.

To enable more flexible therapeutic training, especially for performing daily activities, lightweight and wearable exoskeletons have gained increasing attention. Compared to end-effector-based and grounded exoskeletons, wearable ones can not only provide rehabilitation training anytime/anywhere but also enable personal assistance. However, limited by the size of motors and power supply, current wearable exoskeletons focus on fewer DoFs, such as the flexion of elbow/wrist joint and hand opening/closing. In addition, wearable devices may generate less torque and force on the upper-limb joints. The top row of Fig. 5.3 lists several successful commercialized wearable exoskeletons. MyoPro (AxioBionics, Michigan, US) uses surface EMG sensors to detect the movement intention of users with physical

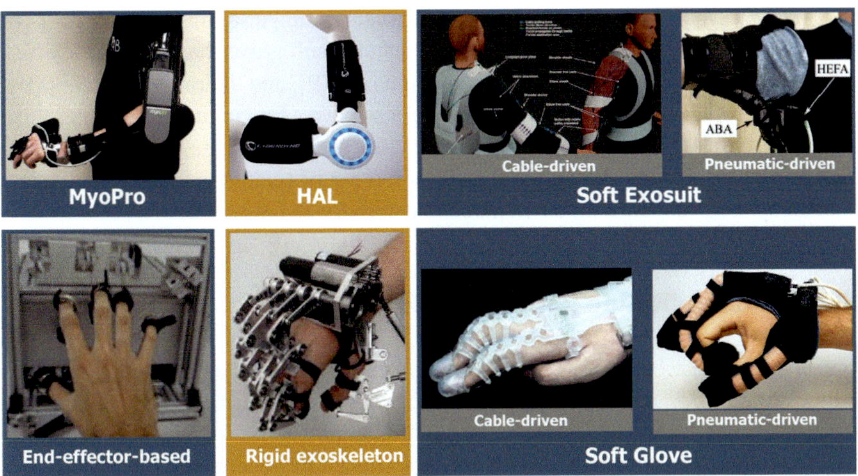

Fig. 5.3 Wearable exoskeletons for upper limb and hand rehabilitation. The upper row demonstrates several wearable exoskeletons for upper limb rehabilitation. For example, MyoPro (AxioBionics, Michigan, US) (adapted with Springer Nature permission from [13]) and HAL (CYBERDYNE, Japan; copyright by CYBERDYNE Inc.) are commercialized rigid exoskeletons for aiding the movement of the elbow joint. Soft exosuits are mainly composed of the cable-driven (adapted from [14] (CC BY 4.0)) or pneumatic-driven (adapted with IEEE permission from [15]) design. Robots for hand rehabilitation including end-effector-based robots (adapted with IEEE permission from [16]), rigid exoskeletons (adapted from [17] (CC BY 4.0)), and soft gloves (adapted with IEEE and Elsevier permissions from [18, 19]) are presented in the lower part

impairment and then assists the flexion of the elbow and wrist as well as hand grasping. Some customized connections are used to improve the comfort level of wearing.

Recent effort has been focused on soft wearable exosuits, which aim to improve the comfort and portability of wearable robots. Instead of using rigid materials and structures, tendon-driven and pneumatic-driven mechanisms have been extensively explored. A cable-driven exosuit was developed by Samper-Escudero et al. [14] to assist shoulder and elbow flexion, where the actuator box was placed in a bag to ensure wearability. Soft textile pneumatic actuators are used to support the upper arm through shoulder abduction and horizontal flexion/extension [15]. It should be noted that compared to servo motors, the precision and speed of pneumatic actuators can be difficult to achieve in practical applications.

The human hand has the most complicated anatomical structure, which includes 22-DoF of the wrist and five fingers. Hence, the development of robots for hand rehabilitation is challenging. As illustrated in the lower part of Fig. 5.3, early attempts were devoted to end-effector-based robots, which were either enabled by using a similar mechanism as robots for upper limbs or achieved by cable-driven designs. However, these end-effector-based systems typically limit the application scenarios to the rehabilitation of clenched hands and hand weakness [16]. For robots to provide both therapeutic training and personal assistance, rigid exoskeletons and soft gloves were additionally developed. The rigid ones were mainly built using linkages, enabling independent control of each hand joint, from a single finger to multiple fingers [17]. With recent advances in soft robotics [20], wearable soft gloves have emerged, which can be driven by tendon/cable [18, 21], pneumatic [19], and hydraulic actuators. The cable-driven ones are advantageous in using less power for continuous holding force for short periods. The pneumatic-driven soft actuators demonstrated the ability to generate uniform force and support the range of motion of each individual finger but are limited by slow response time compared to cable-driven ones.

5.2.2 Rehabilitation Robot for Gait Training

For people with weakness or impaired physical function of lower limbs, previous studies mainly focus on the development of robots for gait training (i.e., the most frequent movement of lower limbs) [22, 23]. Human gait indicates a person's walking or running patterns, involving the motor control of posture stability, balancing, and limb coordination [24]. Gait is a rhythmic movement that can be segmented by two consensus gait events of the same foot, e.g., heel-strike and toe-off. Typically, the movement of lower limbs has less complexity and RoM compared to that of upper limbs, leading to a relatively simple mechanical design. It should be emphasized that the main challenge of robot-assisted gait training lies in balance maintenance and fall prevention, thus requiring large force and torque for the actuators.

More importantly, different kinds of rehabilitation robots for gait training can be used for patients. For patients who are not able to sit or stand, robots are designed to perform therapeutic training at their bedside. For patients lying on a bed, end-effector-based or wearable robotic systems can lift the lower limbs and guide them to simulate cyclic gait movements [25]. Although only passive training is provided, these robots are beneficial for restoring the motor functions of patients at an early stage, thus speeding up the recovery process.

With the progress of recovery, the end-effector robots can help patients with gait training when they are able to stand and move their legs. More specifically, the feet of the patient are fixed on a pedal, while body weight supporting systems are used to protect the patient from falling. Similarly, the mechanical designs involved in end-effector-based gait training robots are relatively simple and easy to build. In addition, these systems can cater to different patients without constraints. As illustrated in the top row of Fig. 5.4, the most popular end-effector-based gait trainers are Gait Trainer GT-I (Reha-Stim Medtec, Berlin, Germany) [30], LokoHelp (Hocoma, Zurich, Switzerland) [31], and G-EO systems (Reha Technology, Olten, Switzerland) [32], which have been extensively used in clinical scenarios. GT1 was the first gait trainer developed in 2000, which supports users to practice gait-like movement on a treadmill and controls the center of mass in the vertical and horizontal directions. In addition, G-EO systems improved gait training in three modes: level walking, ramp walking, and upstairs/downstairs, where the foot trajectory and pose of the user could be corrected to generate more neutral gait patterns. However, these end-effector-based systems lack the capability to control the knee and hip joints, leading to potential abnormal gait patterns after training.

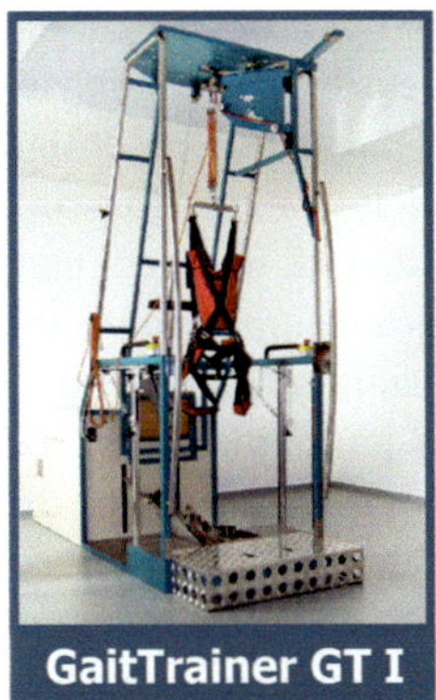

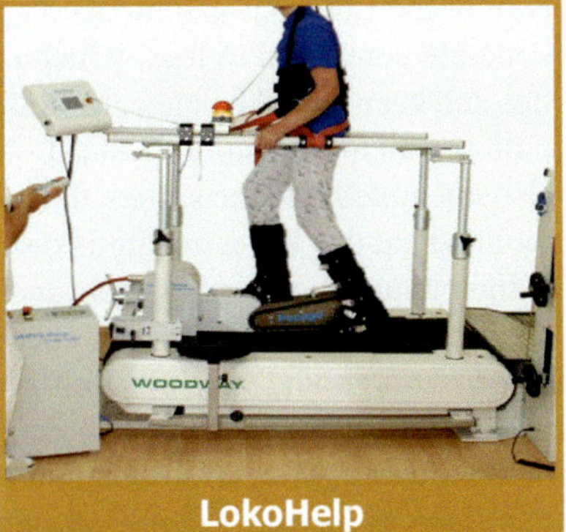

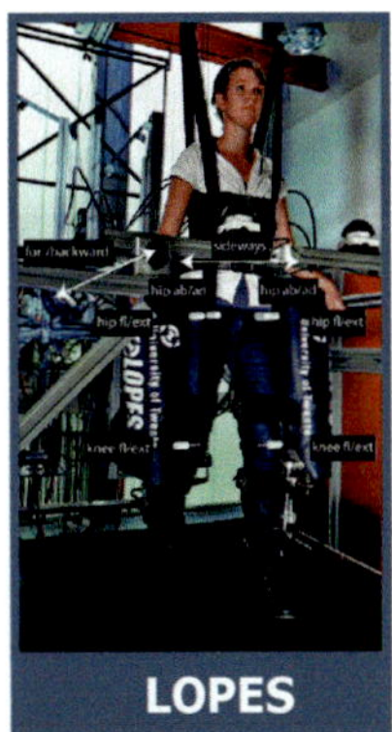

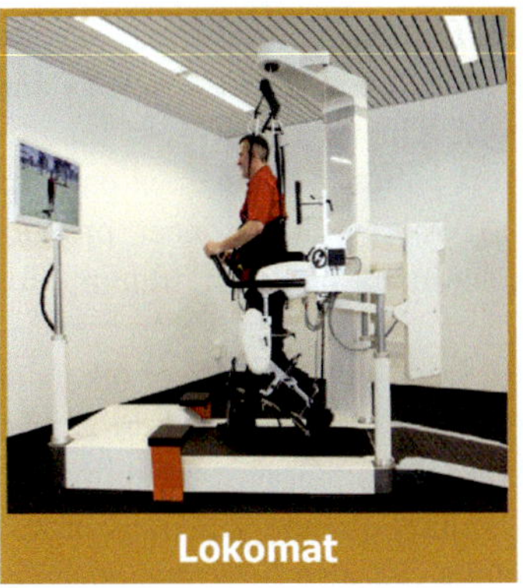

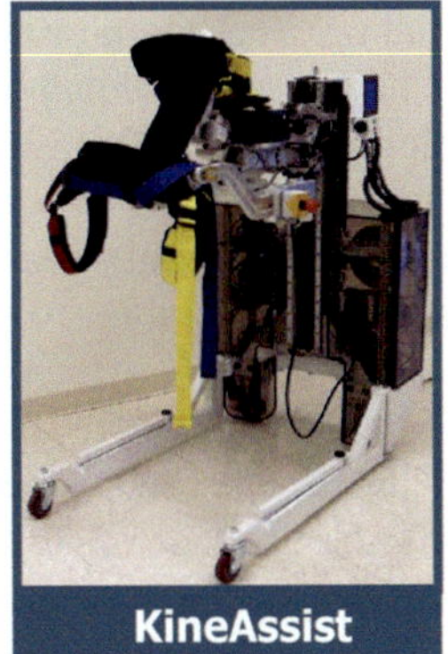

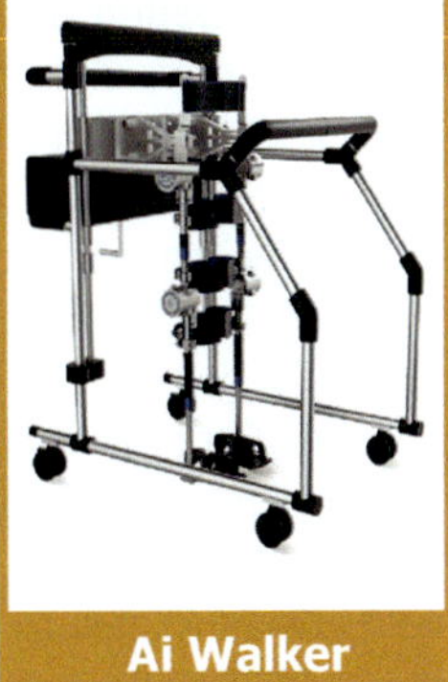

Fig. 5.4 Representative rehabilitation robots for gait training. Two pioneer end-effector-based gait training robots, i.e., Gait Trainer GT-I (Reha-Stim Medtec, Berlin, Germany) (adapted from [26] (CC BY 3.0)) and LokoHelp (Hocoma, Zurich, Switzerland) (adapted from [26] (CC BY 3.0)), are demonstrated in the first row. The treadmill-based exoskeletons for gait rehabilitation, i.e., LOPES [27] (adapted with Springer Nature permission from [28]) and Lokomat (Hocoma, Zurich, Switzerland) (adapted from [26] (CC BY 3.0)) are shown. The exemplar overground gait trainer and robotic walker are listed in the bottom row, including KineAssist (adapted with IEEE permission from [29]) and AiWalker (Ai-Robotics, Beijing, China; copyright by Beijing Ai-Robotics Co. Ltd.)

Consequently, advanced versions of end-effector-based systems were developed, i.e., treadmill-based exoskeletons. On the one hand, these grounded systems use the advantages of end-effector-based systems, where the body weight supporting module can provide compensation for gravity and the use of a treadmill can limit the training in a confined space. On the other hand, the exoskeletons align well with the human bones and are able to aid the motion of each anatomical joint (hip, knee, ankle) individually, which can help make personalized training plans and improve the gait training performance. Popular treadmill-based exoskeletons include LOPES [27] and Lokomat (Hocoma, Zurich, Switzerland) [33], as shown in Fig. 5.4. Lokomat, a well-known grounded exoskeleton for gait training, was developed in 2003. In the past two decades, it has been continuously upgraded and successfully commercialized. The core of the Lokomat system is composed of a multi-DoF hip joint and mechanical structure connected to legs, which can ensure the free movement of lower extremities and keep lateral balance. Moreover, the multi-DoF design allows users to change their walking direction, instead of solely walking forward. Interactive games are also integrated into the system to facilitate task-oriented rehabilitation. It should be pointed out that these treadmill systems are cumbersome and expensive, which limits their applications in hospitals and rehabilitation centers.

It has been shown that there are significant differences in joint kinematics and temporal variables between overground and treadmill walking [34]. Hence, the aforementioned treadmill-based systems may cause unnatural gait after recovery. To overcome these problems, another line of research has focused on the development of overground gait trainers or robotic walkers, encouraging patients to walk on the floor independently. During training, the robotic systems provide either active or passive protection from falling. The bottom row of Fig. 5.4 demonstrates several commercial systems that have been successfully used, i.e., KineAssist [29] and AiWalker (Ai-Robotics, Beijing, China). For example, KineAssist involves a multi-DoF pelvic orthotic structure that can actively correct patients' movement patterns and enable balance training at the same time. AiWalker, the pioneer product launched in China, combines a wearable exoskeleton to facilitate training for patients at different stages.

Even after rehabilitation, when patients are able to walk with the help of others or by themselves, they may still encounter motor weakness or walk with abnormal gait patterns. Consequently, wearable exoskeletons can be an important post-rehabilitation aid. Early exoskeletons were designed primarily for military use and then transformed into healthcare scenarios. These wearable exoskeletons can also help support body weight during sit-to-stand motion and improve balance. Figure 5.5 illustrates several popular wearable exoskeletons for gait training with FDA approval. Ekso, also known

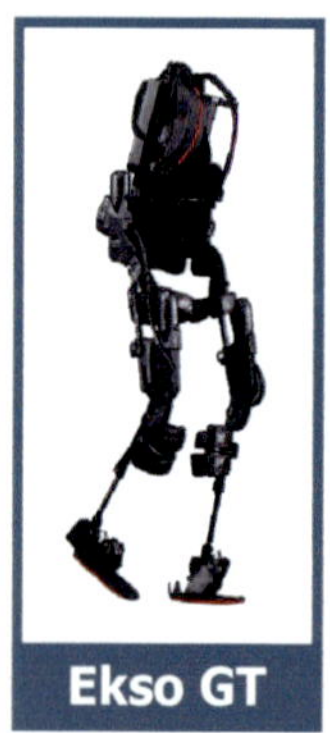

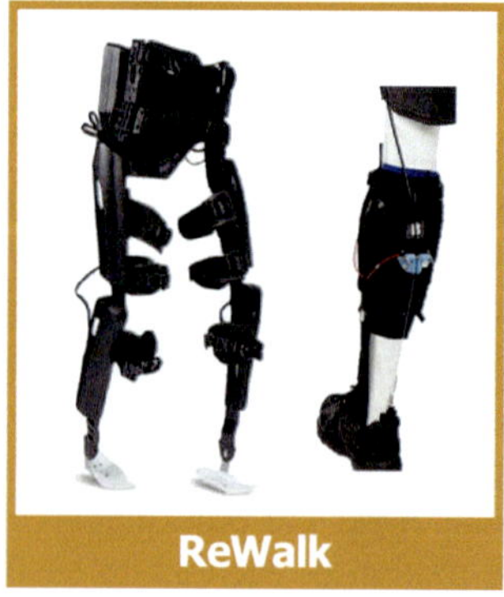

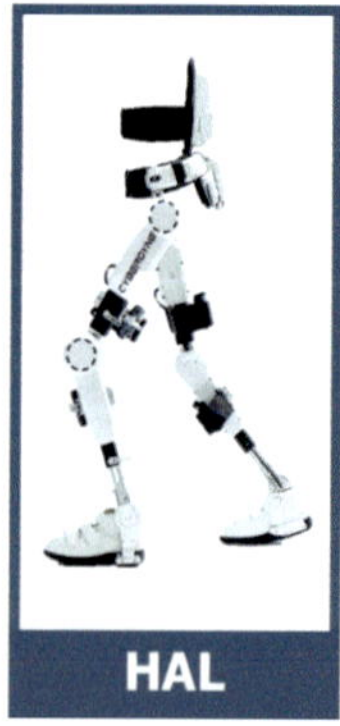

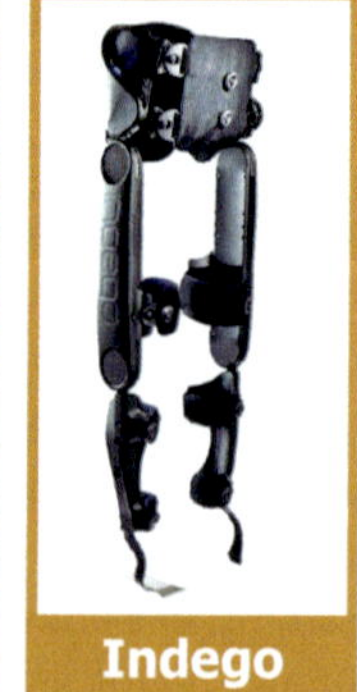

Fig. 5.5 Wearable exoskeletons for gait rehabilitation and walking assistance. They include Ekso GT (Ekso Bionics, Berkeley, US; © 2022 Ekso Bionics), ReWalk Personal/ReStore (ReWalk Robotics Inc., Marlborough, USA; © 2023 ReWalk Robotics), HAL (CYBERDYNE Inc., Tsukuba, Japan; copyright by CYBERDYNE Inc.), Indego (Indego, Vanderbilt University, US; copyright by Indego)

as HULC, produces a wearable bionic exoskeleton developed by Berkeley [35]. In 2016, the Ekso GT™ (Ekso Bionics, Berkeley, US) was the first commercialized exoskeleton cleared by the FDA for rehabilitation use for stroke patients. It allows the adjustment of how much assistance the device gives to each leg. Depending on the mobility of users, they can also use walking sticks to support their body weight and assist with walking. After training with Ekso, the walking speed of patients can be significantly improved. ReWalk Personal™ (ReWalk Robotics Inc., Marlborough, USA) was the first wearable exoskeleton with FDA approval for home and public use [36]. In addition, ReWalk released a soft version called ReStore™, which is the first robotic system with FDA approval for stroke therapy.

Although these wearable exoskeletons have demonstrated effectiveness in walking assistance, the rigid structures inevitably restrict the flexibility and DoFs of lower limb joints (especially for hip and ankle joints). Moreover, rigid exoskeletons are heavy and cumbersome, which may cause collateral trauma when human movement intention is not well interpreted. Recently, different soft lower-limb exoskeletons have gained increasing attention. Conor Walsh and his colleagues from Harvard University initiated the development of a wearable exosuit [22]. They developed a cable-driven soft exosuit to assist the paretic limb of stroke patients and generate forward propulsion to improve their gait patterns [22]. The exosuit is composed of soft materials, thus significantly reducing the weight and increasing the portability. In addition, the cables are aligned with the direction of muscles, which can generate more natural assistance. Based on this exosuit, they further proposed a human-in-the-loop optimization strategy, for which the duration and amplitude of assistance could be varied during walking by minimizing the metabolic energy consumption [37].

5.3 Robots for Personal Assistance

5.3.1 Assistive Robots for ADL

In the past decades, numerous assistive robots have been developed, as illustrated in Fig. 5.6. In this section, we give a brief summary of the commonly used assistive robots.

One of the popular assistive robots is the feeding robot that allows self-feeding for disabled people to support their independence in daily living. For instance, My Spoon (SECOM Co. Ltd., Tokyo, Japan) is a small-size dining assistive robot that enables users to select different control modes, from semi-autonomy to full autonomy. Obi (Desin, US) is also a portable robotic self-feeder for people with upper limb mobility problems, with which the user can self-feed.

In addition, flexible robotic arms have gained increasing popularity in providing personal assistance in daily life. One of the representative assistive robotic arms is Jaco (Kinova, Quebec, Canada) [38, 39], which can be mounted either on the table or on a mobile wheelchair to help with different ADL tasks, e.g., grasping objects, self-feeding, or opening doors. With recent advances in human–robot interaction and robot learning, these robotic arms are able to understand the human intention and perform tasks automatically through voice commands, hand gestures, eye movements, or brain

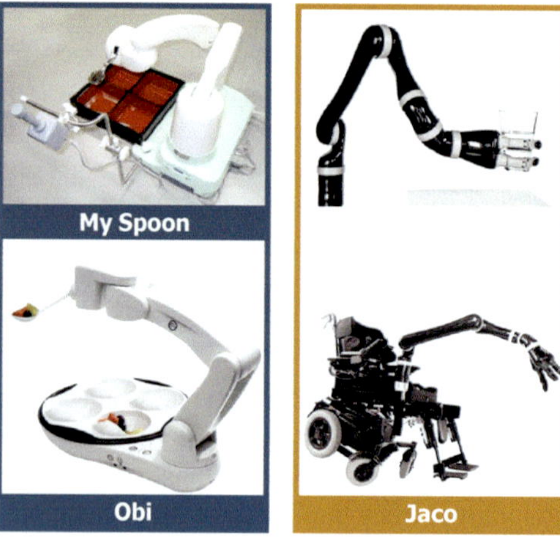

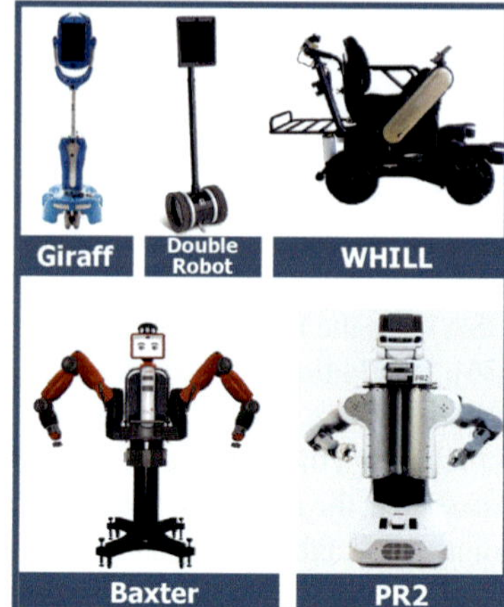

Fig. 5.6 Assistive robots for ADL. Several examples are shown, including feeding robots, assistive robot arms, and mobile assistive robots. Feeding robots: My Spoon (SECOM Co. Ltd., Tokyo, Japan; SECOM Co., Ltd. © 2000–2023) and Obi (Desin, US; Obi, © 2023); assistive robotic arms: Jaco (Kinova, Quebec, Canada; Kinova Inc., © 2023); mobile assistive robots: Giraff (Giraff Technologies AB, Vasteras, Sweden; copyright by Giraff Technologies AB); Double Robot (Double Robotics, Berlin, Germany; Double Robotics, © 2023), WHILL (WHILL, Japan; WHILL Inc., © 2015–2023), Baxter (Rethink Robotics, Bochum, Germany; copyright by Rethink Robotics), and PR2 (Willow Garage, California, US; copyright by Willow Garage)

activities. Meanwhile, advanced computer vision algorithms are incorporated into the robotic system to achieve object detection and recognition.

Another line of research focused on mobile assistive robots. For instance, telepresence robots, e.g., Giraff (Giraff Technologies AB, Vasteras) and Double Robot (Double Robotics, Berlin, Germany), are designed to provide patient monitoring and telemedicine in home-based environments [40]. Integrating with human pose estimation and object detection, these robots can be used to perform gait analysis and fall risk detection at homes [41]. Mobile robots integrated with robotic arms, e.g., Baxter (Rethink Robotics, Bochum, Germany) and PR2 (Willow Garage, California, US), can help people with complex tasks, such as caregiving and dressing [42]. Intelligent wheelchairs represent another type of mobile assistive robot, which can support disabled people navigating freely both at home and in outdoor environments.

5.3.2 Assistive Robots for Human Movement Augmentation

Assistive robots also play significant roles in augmenting human movement. These can either enable humans to perform complicated tasks alone with respect to DoF augmentation or complete specific tasks with less effort in terms of power augmentation [43].

5.3.2.1 Degree-of-Freedom Augmentation

In the past decades, increasing attention has been gained on the development of supernumerary robotics limbs for augmenting human movement with additional DoFs [44]. With the help of supernumerary robotic limbs, users are able to perform complicated tasks alone, which are impossible for bimanual manipulation. Commonly, previous studies were focused on the augmentation of arms [45], fingers [46], and legs [47]. For instance, a third arm allows the user to multitask or help the user to carry an object. While for supernumerary fingers and legs, previous studies mainly focused on the compensation of impaired movement [45]. Through the use of HMIs (e.g., brain signals) or other body interfaces (e.g., foot interface), the control of these extra robotic limbs can be achieved [45, 48].

5.3.2.2 Power Augmentation

Another branch of research on assistive robotics was aimed at increasing human musculoskeletal power, thus enabling users to complete heavy tasks with reduced load or increased speed. In this field, most assistive robots for power augmentation were built on exoskeletons and soft exosuits [49]. When lifting objects, people are at risk of injury by choosing a comfortable posture or lifting heavy objects. To this end, assistive robots for augmenting lifting capability have attracted increasing attention. Cho and his colleagues developed a passive exosuit based on a body-powered variable-impedance mechanism, facilitating squatting rather than stooping [50]. Several robots have been designed to empower human strength using either pneumatic-driven [51] or cable-driven actuators [14].

For lower limbs, lightweight hip/ankle exoskeletons are able to reduce the energy cost during walking and running [52–54], as shown in Fig. 5.7. Collins and his colleagues developed an unpowered ankle exoskeleton by using a ratchet-and-pawl that mechanically engages the spring when the foot is on the ground and disengage it when the foot is in the air [53]. This simple yet effective design can provide some of the functions of the calf muscles and tendons during walking. Recently, they upgraded this robot to both powered and unpowered versions, improving the energy economy during running [54]. By monitoring real-time metabolic consumption,

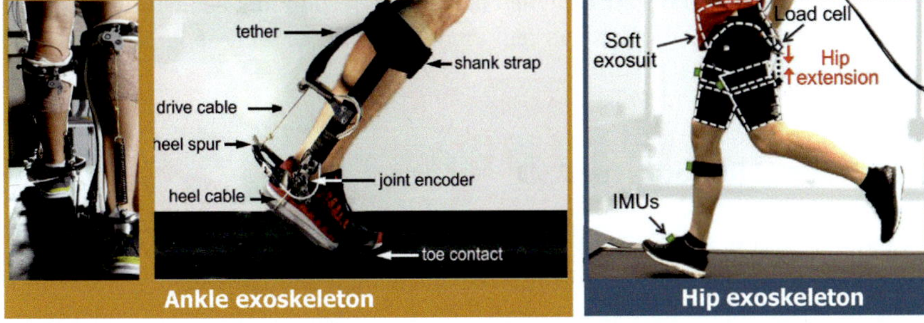

Fig. 5.7 Exoskeletons for augmenting human walking and running. Images are adapted with Nature Publishing Group permission from [53], with AAAS permission from [52, 54]

Walsh et al. from Harvard University introduced a human-in-the-loop strategy for controlling a tethered soft exosuit to assist with hip extension [52].

5.4 Social Robotics for Cognitive Assistance

Social robotics, an emerging research field, is the development of robots that can interact and communicate with humans by following social interaction behaviors [55, 56]. Social robotics is a multidisciplinary research field, which combines robotics, artificial intelligence, sensing, psychology, neuroscience, and social and behavioral science. In recent years, a number of social robots with distinct appearances have been developed, ranging from nonanimal and animal-like to humanoid ones. In recent years, social robotics has gained increasing popularity in healthcare applications, especially for providing social assistance and cognition rehabilitation for people with ASD or dementia [57, 58]. More importantly, social robots integrating multimodal sensing technologies can be deployed at home, thus providing long-term intervention and rehabilitation. In addition, with long-term data collection, the internal relationship between cognition and behavior can be modeled, facilitating the development of personalized intervention and rehabilitation.

The core of social robotics is to realize human-centered social interaction. In daily life, language and human action are the most intuitive representation of behaviors, encoding cognition and interactive intention [59]. Human beings can adjust their social patterns according to each other's emotional states [60]. In addition to facial expressions and language, human behaviors, body language, and physiological signals also imply emotion [61]. Therefore, the understanding of targets' social behaviors and emotion through multimodal perception [such as visual perception, eye tracking, *Electroencephalography* (EEG)] is important in the development of social robots. In other words, it is a prerequisite for social robots to realize human-centered interaction to recognize and predict human action, intention, emotion, perception, and mental state through their posture, gesture, eye contact, and facial expression [62, 63]. Figure 5.8 shows several examples of the interaction between social robots and human subjects. To enable bidirectional interaction between social robots and humans, robots are designed to make corresponding behavioral decisions and express their social behaviors and emotions [55], as well as gain the trust of human users [56].

5.4.1 Social Robotics for ASD

As the biomarkers and specific causes of ASD have not been clearly discovered, early diagnosis and intervention are the main methods for treating ASD [67]. Hitherto, social robots have demonstrated their potential in providing regular interventions for autism patients, trying to improve their eye contact, self-initiated

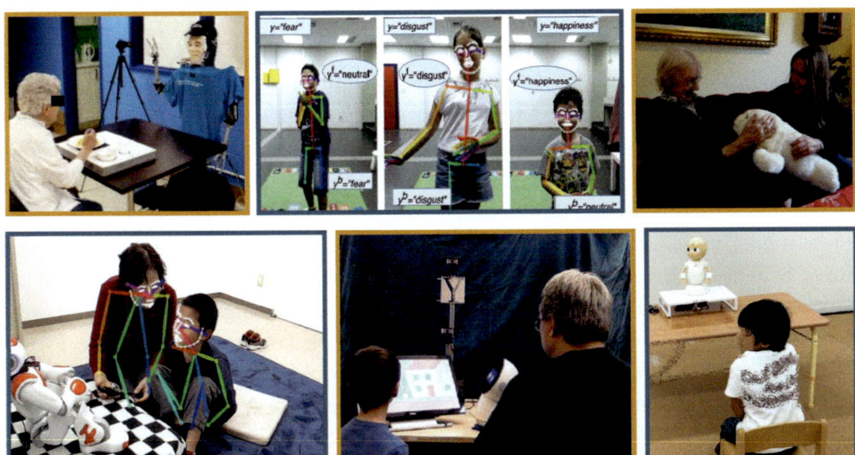

Fig. 5.8 Social robots. Social robots can interact with children with ASD or the elderly with dementia by understanding their movement and cognition behaviors, allowing personalized rehabilitation and intervention treatment in different scenarios. Top row: Images are adapted with ACM permission from [62], with IEEE permission from [63], and under CC BY 4.0 license. Bottom row: Images are adapted with AAAS permissions from [64, 65], and adapted from [66] under CC BY 4.0 license

interactions, turn-taking activities, imitation, emotion recognition, joint attention, and triadic interaction [57, 68, 69].

Joint attention based on social robots is a popular behavioral intervention in previous ASD studies, in which eye-tracking techniques play significant roles in capturing the point of gaze of the targets. Scassellati and colleagues from Yale University explored the use of social robots in the home environment with a 1-month intervention for each ASD child [65]. Using six well-designed interactive games, the social robot interacted with the participants and caregivers for 30 min a day. The experimental results showed that after interacting with the social robot for a period of time, the joint attention of the child and the caregiver were both significantly improved, suggesting the feasibility and effectiveness of the robot for the cultivation of social skills in ASD children. It has also been shown that ASD patients pay more attention to the faces of robots rather than human faces [70].

Due to the intrinsic discrepancy across subjects, previous studies suggested that the detection of emotion and engagement using personalized models can facilitate the interaction between ASD patients and social robots [64, 71]. Rudovic et al. investigated personalized machine learning algorithms to model the interaction between ASD children and social robots, proving the feasibility of using robots to assess the therapeutic effect and engagement of autistic children [64]. By integrating visual data captured from robots and wearable sensing data, the proposed network achieved nearly 60% accuracy in evaluating the treatment effect, mood, and engagement of children with autism.

5.4.2 Social Robotics for Dementia

For patients with dementia, social robots can not only increase their independence but also assist in therapy sessions. More importantly, social robots play a major role in companionship, which have been demonstrated to be effective in reducing tensions between patients and caregivers. Based on a number of observational studies on the therapeutic effects of interaction between patients with Alzheimer's disease and different robots, animal-like robots have shown effectiveness in improving the quality of life of patients with dementia [58, 72]. These cute animal-like robots can increase the happiness and calm of patients in a natural way, while reducing agitation and anxiety. Research also demonstrated that after a long-term accompaniment by the PARO robot, the mood and behavior in dementia patients could be modulated [72].

In addition, humanoid social robots have also been used. By demonstrating specific postures and actions to patients, these robots can guide patients to imitate the robot's movement, thus achieving physical therapy [73]. Moreover, robots can give feedback by using facial expressions or speeches, enhancing the engagement of patients. Humanoid robots were also used to guide the food intake of people with dementia [62]. Another line of research focuses on telepresence robots built on mobile platforms. These kinds of robots are capable of monitoring patients remotely [74].

5.5 Prostheses

For human movement, online commands are first generated by brain cortices, then transmitted to skeletal muscles through the spinal cord, and finally the desired movement is completed by hands or limbs. The sensory information (e.g., tactile, visual, auditory) provides feedback to the brain to close the loop. For amputees or paralyzed patients, the aforementioned bidirectional link cannot be formed due to the loss of body parts or missing functions. Hence, intelligent prosthetics aim to compensate for the lost physical functions and rebuild the sensory feedback of the human body [75], thus performing ADL by receiving their online commands [76].

The development of prosthetics started several centuries ago, and the conventional passive hook-like prosthetic hands represent simple, early embodiments. In the 1960s, "Russia hand" was regarded as the first active prosthetic hand, and Ottobock launched the first commercial product driven by myoelectrical signals. Compared to conventional passive prostheses, active ones can be driven by the intention of users through multimodal interfaces, thus allowing them to perform complex and multifunctional movements [77]. With recent advances in mechatronics and materials, the development of anthropomorphic and dexterous prosthetics is on the rise [78]. Figure 5.9 demonstrates several successful commercial prosthetics, from bionic hands to prosthetic limbs.

In the field of intelligent prosthetics, a commonly used framework is that a human motion intention is first decoded from either brain signals or muscle activities through different HMIs [77]. Then, dedicated control algorithms taking the online commands are executed to generate the movement of the prostheses [79].

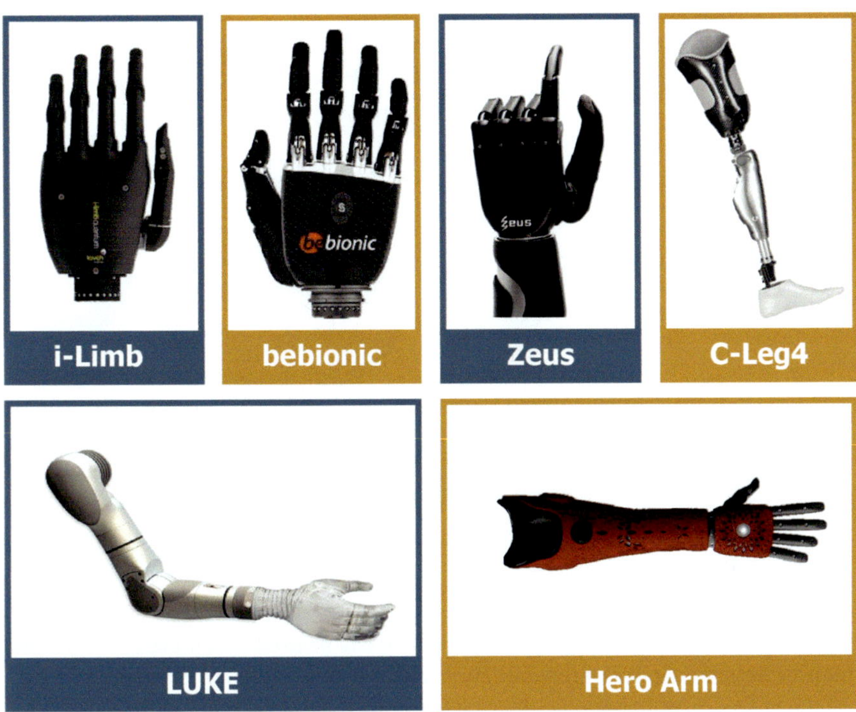

Fig. 5.9 Commercialized prostheses. Several commercialized prostheses are demonstrated, including i-Limb hand (Össur, Reykjavik, Iceland; Össur, © 2023); bebionic hand and C-Leg4 (Ottobock, Minnesota, US; copyright by Ottobock); Zeus hand (Aether Biomedical, Poznan, Poland; Aether Biomedical, © 2023); LUKE arm (Mobius Bionics, Manchester, UK; Mobius Bionics, © 2023); Hero Arm (Open Bionics, Bristol, UK; Open Bionics, © 2022)

Moreover, the prostheses are integrated with different sensors to capture multimodal information. Such information is translated into signals and then stimulates corresponding neurons or muscles to generate sensory feedback [75, 80].

In addition, several studies explored the combination of hip exoskeleton with prosthetic legs, aiming to improve performance and reduce the metabolic cost during walking [81]. In the following section, we will provide more details on human–robot interaction and human–machine interfaces for robot control and sensory feedback.

5.6 Human–Robot Interaction

Human–Robot Interaction (HRI) is a critical part of rehabilitation and assistive robotics, which can construct the bidirectional communication between a human and a robot, and additionally enable human-in-the-loop control of robots [82]. For the human-to-robot session, the human intention is then perceived from different

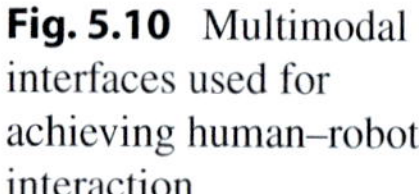

Fig. 5.10 Multimodal interfaces used for achieving human–robot interaction

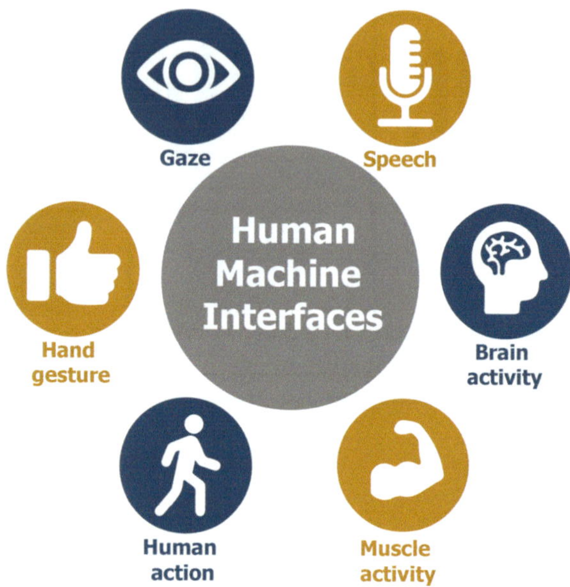

HMIs, as shown in Fig. 5.10. Such information can be used to achieve real-time and intuitive forward control of rehabilitation and assistive robots. In terms of the robot-to-human feedforward session, the robots transmit the perceptual information back to the human, thus closing the loop of the bidirectional interaction. Different types of sensory feedback techniques have been explored to transmit the perceived information back to humans through embodied HMI.

5.6.1 Multimodal Interfaces for HRI

Table 5.1 summarizes the most popular sensing modalities that were used for enabling real-time and reliable HRI, including the detection of muscle activities, brain activities, and visual information.

5.6.1.1 Muscle Interfaces

EMG generated by muscle activities has been widely used in rehabilitation and assistive robotics, especially for active prosthetic control [83]. Due to its wearability and portability, noninvasive *surface EMG* (sEMG) can be measured by attaching sensors to the skin. Extensive research has explored sEMG with different channels, sensor positions, and amputations [84]. To acquire sufficient information on motion intention, high-density sEMG was developed by using a spatially distributed two-dimensional electrode array. However, electrical signals collected from sEMG are easily contaminated by noise and cross-talk effects [85]. Alternatively, invasive *intramuscular EMG* (iEMG) records the electrical signals through needles or wires inserted into muscles, which can

Table 5.1 Different sensing modalities that form the human–machine interface

Interface	Modality	Information
Muscle interface	surface Electromyography (sEMG)	Electrical signals induced by muscle contraction
	intramuscular Electromyography (iEMG)	Electrical signals induced by muscle contraction
	Sonomyography (SMG)	Ultrasonic data of muscle contraction
	Mechanomyography (MMG)	Mechanical response of muscle
Brain interface	Electroencephalography (EEG)	Electrical signals on the scalp
	Electrocorticography (ECoG)	Electrical signals from the cerebral cortex
	functional Near-Infrared Spectroscopy (fNIRS)	Cortical hemodynamic activity
	functional MRI (fMRI)	Cortical hemodynamic activity
	Magnetoencephalography (MEG)	Magnetic fields associated with neural electrical activity
Visual interface	Gaze/eye movement	Visual attention and cognition
	Egocentric vision	Visual information from first-person view
	Electrooculography (EOG)	Electrical signals between the cornea and Bruch's membrane
Other	Voice	Human speech
	Physiological signals	Heart rate, metabolic consumption, respiration

ensure stable and reliable connection and data acquisition. In addition to EMG, *Sonomyography* (SMG) and *Mechanomyography* (MMG) were also used to measure muscle activities [84]. SMG leverages ultrasound imaging techniques to measure morphological changes in the contraction of muscles, while MMG collects the mechanical vibrations of muscles through microphones or vibrometers, which can be further used to infer force and kinematics.

5.6.1.2 Brain–Machine Interface

Human brain activities encode sufficient information on motion intention, especially for neurons in the motor cortex. In recent years, *Brain–Machine Interface* (BMI) or *Brain–Computer Interface* (BCI) has gained increasing popularity in establishing effective interfaces [86]. *Electrocorticography* (ECoG) directly measures the electrical activities of cortical neurons through the implanted electrode arrays attached to the surface of the cerebral cortex [87]. Although invasive, this can collect brain signals with high quality and high spatial resolution, especially for decoding fine-grade movement intention for prosthetic control [88]. However, these invasive devices require complicated surgical procedures for implantation, bringing safety and biocompatibility issues as well. EEG is a noninvasive mechanism to measure cerebral electrophysiological activities from the surface of the scalp, allowing data to be captured in a portable and convenient manner. In the field of rehabilitation and assistive robotics, EEG-based techniques (e.g., motor imagery and steady-state visually evoked potential) are widely used for HRI [89]. Recently, *functional Near-Infrared Spectroscopy* (fNIRS) has been used to detect oxygenation levels and estimate the hemodynamic activity of the brain. This has high spatial resolution compared to EEG. Additionally, with the rapid progress of real-time neuroimaging, *functional MRI* (fMRI) and *Magnetoencephalogram* (MEG) can also be used for BMI.

5.6.1.3 Visual Interfaces

Visual perception is one of the most important sensory channels that receives information from the outside world. It not only encodes human visual attention and motion intention but also involves human cognition and emotion [90]. Recent advances in eye-tracking techniques allow accurate and real-time gaze information of the target person. In addition, an egocentric vision that perceives visual attention from the first-person viewpoint also encodes similar information. Such visual cues can either provide intuitive control signals based on intentions perceived from high-level image sequences or help generate natural and dexterous manipulations for hand–eye coordination based on the shape and pose of target objects [21, 91]. Current commercially available wearable eye-tracking glasses allow simultaneous collection of both gaze behaviors and egocentric vision. In addition, *Electrooculography* (EOG) is a technique for measuring the electrical signals between the cornea and Bruch's membrane and then inferring the movement of eyeballs. Commonly, EOG is used along with EEG to form the HMI for robot control [89].

5.6.2 HRI for Robot Control

Rehabilitation and assistive robots are closely connected to human bodies, allowing the collaboration of robots and human beings in therapeutic training and personal assistance. Hence, the development of an appropriate robot control strategy is a critical topic in rehabilitation and assistive robotics, enabling human–robot interaction in a safe, natural, comfortable, and intelligent manner.

5.6.2.1 Robot Control Strategies

For rehabilitation purposes, different control strategies have been proposed in previous studies. The control strategy of a rehabilitation robot generally follows a hierarchical manner, where impedance and admittance control algorithms are utilized to achieve passive and active modes. Another way to balance the tradeoff between active and passive modes is the assist-as-needed control strategy. In addition, game theory has also gained increasing popularity in designing control algorithms for versatile physical human–robot interaction.

For prosthetic control, current cognition and decision algorithms embedded in the prosthetic controller are based on offline training, and they require training or calibration first. Moreover, the fatigue caused by long-term use and accumulated cognition burden could also affect signal characteristics. To mitigate potential bias and facilitate seamless control, online adaptive algorithms, such as meta-learning and online transfer learning, can be taken into account. A combination of complementary information extracted from multiple modalities could enhance the precision and intuitiveness of prosthetic control. It could also potentially facilitate a more natural control of complex movements.

5.6.2.2 Myoelectric Control Scheme

Myoelectric signals have been widely used for controlling rehabilitation and assistive robots, especially for prosthetic control [92]. A direct strategy is the dual-site control of robots based on signals from antagonistic muscle pairs, where the motor speed is determined by the amputation of the EMG signals. In addition, additional DoFs are controlled by the co-contraction of muscle pairs. However, these direct strategies involve considerable training and careful determination of patient-specific thresholds, leading to a low generalization capability to other users. With multichannel EMG acquisition, the spatiotemporal features extracted from various learning-based methods can be used for recognizing different patterns for complex motion control. With more informative data collected by either iEMG or high-density EMG, complex movements can be decoded, potentially addressing the challenging prediction tasks in rehabilitation robots and prosthetic control [93]. With recent advancements in artificial intelligence, more accurate real-time dexterous movement (e.g., the movement of each individual finger) can be inferred from myoelectric signals [94].

5.6.2.3 BCI-Based Mind Control

Existing BCI-based control methods are either based on motor imagery or external stimuli [95]. Motor imagery indicates that a subject imagines a movement without actually performing it, where the related brain activities can be used as the control commands for the robots. The most frequently used one in motor imagery is *Sensorimotor Rhythm* (SMR), where the amplitude of rhythmic activity within SMR decreases while increasing motion imagery and increases while relaxing, denoted as *Event-Related Desynchronization* (ERD) and *Event-Related Synchronization* (ERS) regulation, respectively. Extensive studies have been conducted to leverage ERD/ERS for decoding human motion intention [96, 97]. However, it remains challenging to predict kinematics from SMR-based BCI, impeding intuitive and natural control.

Significant progress has been made through the use of implant electrodes to extract high-density electrical signals from the cerebral cortex, enabling a real-time and accurate estimation of imagined movement [96, 98]. Stimulation-based BCI, on the other hand, tracks the event-related signals induced by an external stimulus (e.g., vision, auditory). Among these, *Steady-State Visual Evoked Potential* (SSVEP) is the most popular paradigm for robot control [99]. Under SSVEP, the visual stimuli flickered at different frequencies are shown to the subjects, who needed to select the correct target in visual stimuli. In this way, the collected EEG signals have a strong correlation with the flickering frequency of the target. Compared to motor imagery-based BCI, SSVEP does not require tedious user training but significantly increases the cognitive load.

5.6.3 HRI for Sensory Feedback

Real-time sensory feedback enabled by HRI can form a closed-loop system for restoring motor functions for rehabilitation purposes [75, 80]. Commonly, visual and auditory systems can provide users with incidental feedback on the robots' speed and position. In addition, the state of the robotic system (e.g., joint torque, joint angles, stiffness) as well as the interactive information with the environment (e.g., tactile and contact force) can be measured and further simulate the sensation of human beings [100, 101]. Such information can be transferred back to the user to compensate for or augment their sensory functions [49, 102], forming a human-in-the-loop mechanism.

5.6.3.1 Homologous Feedback

Homologous feedback delivers the stimulus according to the information received by robots (e.g., a prosthetic hand). Among existing technologies, neural interface techniques, such as peripheral nervous system stimulation and central nervous system stimulation, are mostly used for prosthetic control [103–105]. These methods are achieved by using implanted electrodes or needles to generate stimulation. For instance, electrical brain stimulation on the somatosensory cortex related to the hand region can synchronize the user with a touch sensation on the artificial hand [104]. For the peripheral nervous system, both extralineural and intralineural electrodes can be used to stimulate tactile sensation [105]. However, these invasive electrical stimulations may cause collateral trauma for users. In addition, mechano-tactile stimulation is a noninvasive mechanism of haptic feedback in prostheses, which aims to generate the force perpendicularly when a force is sensed by the prosthetic hand [106]. After training, both amputees and healthy subjects are able to identify the stimulus locations and pressure levels.

5.6.3.2 Sensory Substitution Feedback

Sensory substitution provides feedback in a different form, such as electrotactile and vibrotactile feedback. Electrotactile feedback delivers electrical stimulation to nerve endings through the skin interface [107]. Evidence showed that electrotactile feedback could be used to simulate the sense of slip and pressure, thus improving grasping performance [108]. On the other hand, vibrotactile feedback generates vibrations to simulate tactile sensation, where the frequency, duration, and amplitude of the vibration can be modulated. In addition, auditory stimulation can act as another substitute for tactile feedback.

5.6.3.3 Biofeedback

Biofeedback represents a mechanism where biomechanical and physiological signals measured from different HMIs are delivered back to users via visual, acoustic, or somatosensory manners, helping them learn how their bodies work [109]. With biofeedback, patients are able to automatically change/correct their movement patterns, thus enhancing engagement. This simple yet effective mechanism has demonstrated great potential in rehabilitation training, establishing a "closed control loop" for human subjects. Biomechanical signals include the posture, inertial, force, and pressure of the human body measured by the robotic system, which has been extensively used in previous robot-assisted therapeutic training [110]. However, patients may not easily understand such biomechanical signals.

Signals of neuromuscular and cardiovascular systems are commonly used as physiological biofeedback, in which EMG data indicating the muscle activations offer more intuitive feedback in rehabilitation. In addition, the biofeedback of brain activity is well known as neurofeedback [111], where brain signals measured from EEG or fNIRS have been extensively explored in previous studies. Recently, advanced assistive devices, such as virtual reality and augmented reality, were integrated into robotic rehabilitation systems to provide an immersive way for rehabilitation training with biofeedback mechanisms [112], which can enhance the engagement of patients and guide them to practice in a controlled environment.

5.6.4 HRI for Rehabilitation Assessment

In clinical practice, the motor and cognitive functions are quantitatively evaluated through observation-based clinical scales. However, such assessments heavily rely on the subjective decisions of therapists. Consequently, the objective and quantitative assessment achieved by HRI is another significant topic in robot-assisted therapeutic training.

5.6.4.1 Assessment from Kinematics & Kinetics

One common way of kinematic or kinetic assessment is the use of inertial sensors attached to the robots to measure the kinematic parameters such as motion trajectory, speed, and acceleration of a specific task performed by patients [113]. These are able to quantify movement accuracy, efficiency, inter-limb coordination, and so on. Joint force and torque are kinetic-based indices for assessing abnormal synergies [114]. In previous research, evidence has shown that there is a strong correlation between kinematics/kinetics and clinical assessment scales, which could help understand the process of recovery.

5.6.4.2 Vision-Based Assessment

In order to fully characterize human movement, visual systems have demonstrated their advantages in assessing the compensation of patients and providing feedback for correcting their movement [115]. Different from conventional marker-based motion capture systems, recent advanced markerless human pose estimation can achieve real-time posture assessment and compensation detection during therapeutic training, which is useful to provide feedback to users in real time.

5.6.4.3 Assessment from Muscle and Brain Activities

In practice, there is also a need to evaluate the motor and neurological recovery from patients' muscle and brain activities. sEMG was used in previous studies, where the activation and co-contraction levels are popular indices for assessing recovery [116]. The assessment of brain activities has also gained increasing popularity, where the quantitative measures derived from EEG signals can be used to evaluate both motor and cognitive functions. For instance, EEG signals have been used to model mental engagement and fatigue during therapeutic training [117, 118].

5.7 Conclusions

In this chapter, we have provided an overview of the technical aspects of available robotic systems for therapeutic training, personal assistance, cognitive assistance, prosthetics, and human–robot interaction. For therapeutic training, robotic systems have evolved from conventional grounded robots to the current wearable and portable ones, which aim to provide repetitive and personalized training for patients. Assistive robots are designed to help people manage ADLs or restore lost functions, either physical or perceptual. Nowadays, social robots for cognitive assistive have also emerged, offering personalized care and treatment for those with neurological degradation disease. Prosthetics are typically designed for compensating physical functions of amputees, where bidirectional human–robot interaction plays an important role in forming effective control. In this chapter, we also include a detailed discussion of current human–robot interaction techniques in the field of rehabilitation and assistive robotics. Based on multimodal interfaces, HRI is an effective tool for robot control, sensory feedback, and rehabilitation assessment.

References

1. Yang G-Z, Riener R, Dario P. To integrate and to empower: robots for rehabilitation and assistance. Am Assoc Adv Sci. 2017;2:eaan5593.
2. Chang WH, Kim YH. Robot-assisted therapy in stroke rehabilitation. J Stroke. 2013;15(3):174–81.
3. Tejima N. Rehabilitation robotics: a review. Adv Robot. 2001;14(7):551–64.
4. Krebs HI, Hogan N, Aisen ML, et al. Robot-aided neurorehabilitation. IEEE Trans Rehabil Eng. 1998;6(1):75–87.
5. Molteni F, Gasperini G, Cannaviello G, et al. Exoskeleton and end-effector robots for upper and lower limbs rehabilitation: narrative review. PM&R. 2018;10(9):S174–S88.
6. Poggensee KL, Collins SH. How adaptation, training, and customization contribute to benefits from exoskeleton assistance. Sci Robot. 2021;6(58):eabf1078.

7. Hidler J, Nichols D, Pelliccio M, et al. Advances in the understanding and treatment of stroke impairment using robotic devices. Top Stroke Rehabil. 2005;12(2):22–35.
8. Nef T, Mihelj M, Riener R. ARMin: a robot for patient-cooperative arm therapy. Med Biol Eng Comput. 2007;45(9):887–900.
9. Keller U, Schölch S, Albisser U, et al. Robot-assisted arm assessments in spinal cord injured patients: a consideration of concept study. PLoS One. 2015;10(5):e0126948.
10. Gijbels D, Lamers I, Kerkhofs L, et al. The Armeo spring as training tool to improve upper limb functionality in multiple sclerosis: a pilot study. J Neuroeng Rehabil. 2011;8(1):1–8.
11. Zimmermann Y, Forino A, Riener R, et al. ANYexo: a versatile and dynamic upper-limb rehabilitation robot. IEEE Robot Automat Lett. 2019;4(4):3649–56.
12. Lo HS, Xie SQ. Exoskeleton robots for upper-limb rehabilitation: state of the art and future prospects. Med Eng Phys. 2012;34(3):261–8.
13. Nelson A, Sampson B, Maldonado AA. Prosthetics and orthotics in brachial plexus injury: background, historical perspective, and role of amputation and prosthetic fitting. In: Shin AY, Pulos N, editors. Operative brachial plexus surgery: clinical evaluation and management strategies. Cham: Springer; 2021. p. 417–26.
14. Samper-Escudero JL, Giménez-Fernandez A, Sánchez-Urán MÁ, et al. A cable-driven exosuit for upper limb flexion based on fibres compliance. IEEE Access. 2020;8:153297–310.
15. O'Neill CT, Phipps NS, Cappello L, et al. A soft wearable robot for the shoulder: design, characterization, and preliminary testing. In: Proceedings of the 2017 international conference on rehabilitation robotics (ICORR). IEEE; 2017.
16. Dovat L, Lambercy O, Gassert R, et al. HandCARE: a cable-actuated rehabilitation system to train hand function after stroke. IEEE Trans Neural Syst Rehabil Eng. 2008;16(6):582–91.
17. Troncossi M, Mozaffari-Foumashi M, Parenti-Castelli V. An original classification of rehabilitation hand exoskeletons. J Robot Mech Eng Res. 2016;1(4):17–29.
18. Kang BB, Lee H, In H, et al. Development of a polymer-based tendon-driven wearable robotic hand. In: Proceedings of the 2016 IEEE international conference on robotics and automation (ICRA). IEEE; 2016.
19. Polygerinos P, Wang Z, Galloway KC, et al. Soft robotic glove for combined assistance and at-home rehabilitation. Robot Auton Syst. 2015;73:135–43.
20. Rus D, Tolley MT. Design, fabrication and control of soft robots. Nature. 2015;521(7553):467–75.
21. Kim D, Kang BB, Kim KB, et al. Eyes are faster than hands: a soft wearable robot learns user intention from the egocentric view. Sci Robot. 2019;4(26):eaav2949.
22. Awad LN, Bae J, O'Donnell K, et al. A soft robotic exosuit improves walking in patients after stroke. Sci Transl Med. 2017;9(400):eaai9084.
23. Lerner ZF, Damiano DL, Bulea TC. A lower-extremity exoskeleton improves knee extension in children with crouch gait from cerebral palsy. Sci Transl Med. 2017;9(404):eaam9145.
24. Deligianni F, Guo Y, Yang G-Z. From emotions to mood disorders: a survey on gait analysis methodology. IEEE J Biomed Health Inform. 2019;23(6):2302–16.
25. Ren Y, Wu Y-N, Yang C-Y, et al. Developing a wearable ankle rehabilitation robotic device for in-bed acute stroke rehabilitation. IEEE Trans Neural Syst Rehabil Eng. 2016;25(6):589–96.
26. Díaz I, Gil JJ, Sánchez E. Lower-limb robotic rehabilitation: literature review and challenges. J Robot. 2011;2011:759764.
27. Veneman JF, Kruidhof R, Hekman EE, et al. Design and evaluation of the LOPES exoskeleton robot for interactive gait rehabilitation. IEEE Trans Neural Syst Rehabil Eng. 2007;15(3):379–86.
28. van Asseldonk EH, van der Kooij H. Robot-aided gait training with LOPES. In: Dietz V, Nef T, Rymer W, editors. Neurorehabilitation technology. London: Springer; 2012. p. 379–96.
29. Peshkin M, Brown DA, Santos-Munné JJ, et al. KineAssist: a robotic overground gait and balance training device. In: Proceedings of the 9th international conference on rehabilitation robotics, 2005 (ICORR 2005). IEEE; 2005.

30. Hesse S, Uhlenbrock D. A mechanized gait trainer for restoration of gait. J Rehabil Res Dev. 2000;37(6):701–8.
31. Freivogel S, Mehrholz J, Husak-Sotomayor T, et al. Gait training with the newly developed 'LokoHelp'-system is feasible for non-ambulatory patients after stroke, spinal cord and brain injury. A feasibility study. Brain Inj. 2008;22(7–8):625–32.
32. Hesse S, Waldner A, Tomelleri C. Innovative gait robot for the repetitive practice of floor walking and stair climbing up and down in stroke patients. J Neuroeng Rehabil. 2010;7(1):1–10.
33. Jezernik S, Colombo G, Keller T, et al. Robotic orthosis lokomat: a rehabilitation and research tool. Neuromodulation. 2003;6(2):108–15.
34. Alton F, Baldey L, Caplan S, et al. A kinematic comparison of overground and treadmill walking. Clin Biomech. 1998;13(6):434–40.
35. Angold HKR, Harding N, Richmond K, et al. Ekso bionics-Ekso bionics. IEEE Spectr. 2015;49(1):30–2.
36. Esquenazi A, Talaty M, Packel A, et al. The ReWalk powered exoskeleton to restore ambulatory function to individuals with thoracic-level motor-complete spinal cord injury. Am J Phys Med Rehabil. 2012;91(11):911–21.
37. Ding Y, Kim M, Kuindersma S, et al. Human-in-the-loop optimization of hip assistance with a soft exosuit during walking. Sci Robot. 2018;3(15):eaar5438.
38. Al-Halimi RK, Moussa M. Performing complex tasks by users with upper-extremity disabilities using a 6-DOF robotic arm: a study. IEEE Trans Neural Syst Rehabil Eng. 2016;25(6):686–93.
39. Fall CL, Quevillon F, Blouin M, et al. A multimodal adaptive wireless control interface for people with upper-body disabilities. IEEE Trans Biomed Circuits Syst. 2018;12(3):564–75.
40. Moyle W, Jones C, Cooke M, et al. Connecting the person with dementia and family: a feasibility study of a telepresence robot. BMC Geriatr. 2014;14(1):1–11.
41. Guo Y, Deligianni F, Gu X, et al. 3-D canonical pose estimation and abnormal gait recognition with a single RGB-D camera. IEEE Robot Automat Lett. 2019;4(4):3617–24.
42. Zhang F, Demiris Y. Learning garment manipulation policies toward robot-assisted dressing. Sci Robot. 2022;7(65):eabm6010.
43. Eden J, Bräcklein M, Ibáñez J, et al. Principles of human movement augmentation and the challenges in making it a reality. Nat Commun. 2022;13(1):1–13.
44. Tong Y, Liu J. Review of research and development of supernumerary robotic limbs. IEEE CAA J Autom Sin. 2021;8(5):929–52.
45. Penaloza CI, Nishio S. BMI control of a third arm for multitasking. Sci Robot. 2018;3(20):eaat1228.
46. Malvezzi M, Iqbal Z, Valigi MC, et al. Design of multiple wearable robotic extra fingers for human hand augmentation. Robotics. 2019;8(4):102.
47. Hao M, Zhang J, Chen K, et al. Supernumerary robotic limbs to assist human walking with load carriage. J Mech Robot. 2020;12(6):061014.
48. Dominijanni G, Shokur S, Salvietti G, et al. The neural resource allocation problem when enhancing human bodies with extra robotic limbs. Nat Mach Intell. 2021;3(10):850–60.
49. Walsh C. Human-in-the-loop development of soft wearable robots. Nat Rev Mater. 2018;3(6):78–80.
50. Yun S-S, Kim K, Ahn J, et al. Body-powered variable impedance: an approach to augmenting humans with a passive device by reshaping lifting posture. Sci Robot. 2021;6(57):eabe1243.
51. Thalman CM, Lam QP, Nguyen PH, et al. A novel soft elbow exosuit to supplement bicep lifting capacity. In: Proceedings of the 2018 IEEE/RSJ international conference on intelligent robots and systems (IROS). IEEE; 2018.
52. Lee G, Kim J, Panizzolo F, et al. Reducing the metabolic cost of running with a tethered soft exosuit. Sci Robot. 2017;2(6):eaan6708.
53. Collins SH, Wiggin MB, Sawicki GS. Reducing the energy cost of human walking using an unpowered exoskeleton. Nature. 2015;522(7555):212–5.
54. Witte KA, Fiers P, Sheets-Singer AL, et al. Improving the energy economy of human running with powered and unpowered ankle exoskeleton assistance. Sci Robot. 2020;5(40):eaay9108.

55. Breazeal C, Dautenhahn K, Kanda T. Social robotics. In: Siciliano B, Khatib O, editors. Springer handbook of robotics. Cham: Springer; 2016. p. 1935–72.
56. Yang G-Z, Dario P, Kragic D. Social robotics—trust, learning, and social interaction. Am Assoc Adv Sci. 2018;3:eaau8839.
57. Pennisi P, Tonacci A, Tartarisco G, et al. Autism and social robotics: a systematic review. Autism Res. 2016;9(2):165–83.
58. Góngora Alonso S, Hamrioui S, de la Torre Díez I, et al. Social robots for people with aging and dementia: a systematic review of literature. Telemed e-Health. 2019;25(7):533–40.
59. Gonzalez MC, Hidalgo CA, Barabasi A-L. Understanding individual human mobility patterns. Nature. 2008;453(7196):779–82.
60. Adolphs R. Cognitive neuroscience of human social behaviour. Nat Rev Neurosci. 2003;4(3):165–78.
61. Rose AM. Human behavior and social processes: an interactionist approach. New York: Routledge; 2013.
62. McColl D, Nejat G. Meal-time with a socially assistive robot and older adults at a long-term care facility. J Hum Robot Interact. 2013;2(1):152–71.
63. Filntisis PP, Efthymiou N, Koutras P, et al. Fusing body posture with facial expressions for joint recognition of affect in child–robot interaction. IEEE Robot Automat Lett. 2019;4(4):4011–8.
64. Rudovic O, Lee J, Dai M, et al. Personalized machine learning for robot perception of affect and engagement in autism therapy. Sci Robot. 2018;3(19):eaao6760.
65. Scassellati B, Boccanfuso L, Huang C-M, et al. Improving social skills in children with ASD using a long-term, in-home social robot. Sci Robot. 2018;3(21):eaat7544.
66. Kumazaki H, Yoshikawa Y, Yoshimura Y, et al. The impact of robotic intervention on joint attention in children with autism spectrum disorders. Mol Autism. 2018;9(1):1–10.
67. Reichow B, Barton EE, Boyd BA, et al. Early intensive behavioral intervention (EIBI) for young children with autism spectrum disorders (ASD): a systematic review. Campbell Syst Rev. 2014;10(1):1–116.
68. Cabibihan J-J, Javed H, Ang M, et al. Why robots? A survey on the roles and benefits of social robots in the therapy of children with autism. Int J Soc Robot. 2013;5(4):593–618.
69. Jouaiti M, Henaff P. Robot-based motor rehabilitation in autism: a systematic review. Int J Soc Robot. 2019;11(5):753–64.
70. Cao W, Song W, Li X, et al. Interaction with social robots: improving gaze toward face but not necessarily joint attention in children with autism spectrum disorder. Front Psychol. 2019;10:1503.
71. Jain S, Thiagarajan B, Shi Z, et al. Modeling engagement in long-term, in-home socially assistive robot interventions for children with autism spectrum disorders. Sci Robot. 2020;5(39):eaaz3791.
72. Shibata T. Therapeutic seal robot as biofeedback medical device: qualitative and quantitative evaluations of robot therapy in dementia care. Proc IEEE. 2012;100(8):2527–38.
73. Rouaix N, Retru-Chavastel L, Rigaud A-S, et al. Affective and engagement issues in the conception and assessment of a robot-assisted psychomotor therapy for persons with dementia. Front Psychol. 2017;8:950.
74. Moyle W, Arnautovska U, Ownsworth T, et al. Potential of telepresence robots to enhance social connectedness in older adults with dementia: an integrative review of feasibility. Int Psychogeriatr. 2017;29(12):1951–64.
75. Raspopovic S, Valle G, Petrini FM. Sensory feedback for limb prostheses in amputees. Nat Mater. 2021;20(7):925–39.
76. Farina D, Amsüss S. Reflections on the present and future of upper limb prostheses. Expert Rev Med Devices. 2016;13(4):321–4.
77. Musallam S, Corneil B, Greger B, et al. Cognitive control signals for neural prosthetics. Science. 2004;305(5681):258–62.
78. Farina D, Aszmann O. Bionic limbs: clinical reality and academic promises. Sci Transl Med. 2014;6(257):257ps12.

79. Srinivasan S, Carty M, Calvaresi P, et al. On prosthetic control: a regenerative agonist-antagonist myoneural interface. Sci Robot. 2017;2(6):eaan2971.
80. Antfolk C, D'Alonzo M, Rosén B, et al. Sensory feedback in upper limb prosthetics. Expert Rev Med Devices. 2013;10(1):45–54.
81. Ishmael MK, Archangeli D, Lenzi T. Powered hip exoskeleton improves walking economy in individuals with above-knee amputation. Nat Med. 2021;27(10):1783–8.
82. Guo Y, Gu X, Yang G-Z. Human–robot interaction for rehabilitation robotics. In: Glauner P, Plugmann P, Lerzynski G, editors. Digitalization in healthcare. Cham: Springer; 2021. p. 269–95.
83. Furui A, Eto S, Nakagaki K, et al. A myoelectric prosthetic hand with muscle synergy-based motion determination and impedance model-based biomimetic control. Sci Robot. 2019;4(31):eaaw6339.
84. Fang Y, Hettiarachchi N, Zhou D, et al. Multi-modal sensing techniques for interfacing hand prostheses: a review. IEEE Sensors J. 2015;15(11):6065–76.
85. de Luca CJ, Gilmore LD, Kuznetsov M, et al. Filtering the surface EMG signal: movement artifact and baseline noise contamination. J Biomech. 2010;43(8):1573–9.
86. Hochberg LR, Serruya MD, Friehs GM, et al. Neuronal ensemble control of prosthetic devices by a human with tetraplegia. Nature. 2006;442(7099):164–71.
87. Silversmith DB, Abiri R, Hardy NF, et al. Plug-and-play control of a brain–computer interface through neural map stabilization. Nat Biotechnol. 2021;39(3):326–35.
88. Thakor NV. Translating the brain-machine interface. Sci Transl Med. 2013;5(210):210ps17.
89. Soekadar S, Witkowski M, Gómez C, et al. Hybrid EEG/EOG-based brain/neural hand exoskeleton restores fully independent daily living activities after quadriplegia. Sci Robot. 2016;1(1):eaag3296.
90. Itti L, Koch C. Computational modelling of visual attention. Nat Rev Neurosci. 2001;2(3):194–203.
91. McMullen DP, Hotson G, Katyal KD, et al. Demonstration of a semi-autonomous hybrid brain–machine interface using human intracranial EEG, eye tracking, and computer vision to control a robotic upper limb prosthetic. IEEE Trans Neural Syst Rehabil Eng. 2013;22(4):784–96.
92. Geethanjali P. Myoelectric control of prosthetic hands: state-of-the-art review. Med Dev. 2016;9:247.
93. Kapelner T, Vujaklija I, Jiang N, et al. Predicting wrist kinematics from motor unit discharge timings for the control of active prostheses. J Neuroeng Rehabil. 2019;16(1):1–11.
94. Luu DK, Nguyen AT, Jiang M, et al. Artificial intelligence enables real-time and intuitive control of prostheses via nerve interface. IEEE Trans Biomed Eng. 2022;69(10):3051–63.
95. Abiri R, Borhani S, Sellers EW, et al. A comprehensive review of EEG-based brain–computer interface paradigms. J Neural Eng. 2019;16(1):011001.
96. Aflalo T, Kellis S, Klaes C, et al. Decoding motor imagery from the posterior parietal cortex of a tetraplegic human. Science. 2015;348(6237):906–10.
97. Meng J, Zhang S, Bekyo A, et al. Noninvasive electroencephalogram based control of a robotic arm for reach and grasp tasks. Sci Rep. 2016;6(1):1–15.
98. Hochberg LR, Bacher D, Jarosiewicz B, et al. Reach and grasp by people with tetraplegia using a neurally controlled robotic arm. Nature. 2012;485(7398):372–5.
99. Sakurada T, Kawase T, Takano K, et al. A BMI-based occupational therapy assist suit: asynchronous control by SSVEP. Front Neurosci. 2013;7:172.
100. Zollo L, Di Pino G, Ciancio AL, et al. Restoring tactile sensations via neural interfaces for real-time force-and-slippage closed-loop control of bionic hands. Sci Robot. 2019;4(27):eaau9924.
101. Wu Y, Liu Y, Zhou Y, et al. A skin-inspired tactile sensor for smart prosthetics. Sci Robot. 2018;3(22):eaat0429.
102. Marasco PD, Hebert JS, Sensinger JW, et al. Neurorobotic fusion of prosthetic touch, kinesthesia, and movement in bionic upper limbs promotes intrinsic brain behaviors. Sci Robot. 2021;6(58):eabf3368.

103. Raspopovic S. Neurorobotics for neurorehabilitation. Science. 2021;373(6555):634–5.
104. Collins KL, Guterstam A, Cronin J, et al. Ownership of an artificial limb induced by electrical brain stimulation. Proc Natl Acad Sci. 2017;114(1):166–71.
105. Clites TR, Carty MJ, Ullauri JB, et al. Proprioception from a neurally controlled lower-extremity prosthesis. Sci Transl Med. 2018;10(443):eaap8373.
106. Shi G, Palombi A, Lim Z, et al. Fluidic haptic interface for mechano-tactile feedback. IEEE Trans Haptics. 2020;13(1):204–10.
107. Shi Y, Wang F, Tian J, et al. Self-powered electro-tactile system for virtual tactile experiences. Sci Adv. 2021;7(6):eabe2943.
108. Xu H, Zhang D, Huegel JC, et al. Effects of different tactile feedback on myoelectric closed-loop control for grasping based on electrotactile stimulation. IEEE Trans Neural Syst Rehabil Eng. 2015;24(8):827–36.
109. Giggins OM, Persson UM, Caulfield B. Biofeedback in rehabilitation. J Neuroeng Rehabil. 2013;10(1):1–11.
110. Stoller O, Waser M, Stammler L, et al. Evaluation of robot-assisted gait training using integrated biofeedback in neurologic disorders. Gait Posture. 2012;35(4):595–600.
111. Sitaram R, Ros T, Stoeckel L, et al. Closed-loop brain training: the science of neurofeedback. Nat Rev Neurosci. 2017;18(2):86–100.
112. Mubin O, Alnajjar F, Jishtu N, et al. Exoskeletons with virtual reality, augmented reality, and gamification for stroke patients' rehabilitation: systematic review. JMIR Rehabil Assist Technol. 2019;6(2):e12010.
113. Nordin N, Xie SQ, Wünsche B. Assessment of movement quality in robot-assisted upper limb rehabilitation after stroke: a review. J Neuroeng Rehabil. 2014;11(1):1–23.
114. Kung P-C, Lin C-CK, Ju M-S. Neuro-rehabilitation robot-assisted assessments of synergy patterns of forearm, elbow and shoulder joints in chronic stroke patients. Clin Biomech. 2010;25(7):647–54.
115. Debnath B, O'Brien M, Yamaguchi M, et al. A review of computer vision-based approaches for physical rehabilitation and assessment. Multimedia Systems. 2022;28:209–39.
116. Hu X, Tong K, Song R, et al. Quantitative evaluation of motor functional recovery process in chronic stroke patients during robot-assisted wrist training. J Electromyogr Kinesiol. 2009;19(4):639–50.
117. Park W, Kwon GH, Kim D-H, et al. Assessment of cognitive engagement in stroke patients from single-trial EEG during motor rehabilitation. IEEE Trans Neural Syst Rehabil Eng. 2014;23(3):351–62.
118. Foong R, Ang KK, Quek C, et al. Assessment of the efficacy of EEG-based MI-BCI with visual feedback and EEG correlates of mental fatigue for upper-limb stroke rehabilitation. IEEE Trans Biomed Eng. 2019;67(3):786–95.

Hospital Automation Robotics

6

Contents

6.1 Introduction

Robots are becoming ubiquitous in healthcare in recent years [1, 2]. To address the increasing demand in clinical applications, we have witnessed the popularity of medical robotics in surgery, rehabilitation, and personal assistance [2–8]. Another important category in medical robotics lies in the development of robotic systems to improve the automation levels of hospitals [9].

As shown in Fig. 6.1, hospital automation robots can assist clinicians in different routine tasks in hospitals, including hospital logistics, pharmacy and drug management, and patient transfer and care. For example, robots for hospital logistics include robotic systems for reception, disinfection, inventory management, and in-hospital delivery. Robots are advantageous in carrying heavy supplies with high efficiency, preventing human workers from potential risks, and dealing with dull and repetitive tasks. Robots working in a pharmacy department could provide error-free pick and place, blend, and dispensing of drugs. To deal with tedious tasks in patient transfer, robots could help move patients from one place to another, and robotic nurses can

Y. Guo et al., *Medical Robotics*, Innovative Medical Devices,
https://doi.org/10.1007/978-981-99-7317-0_6

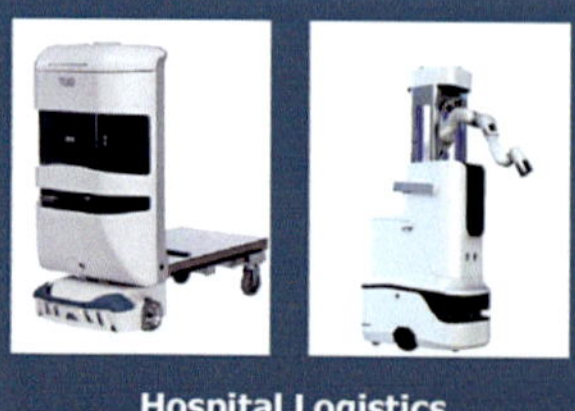

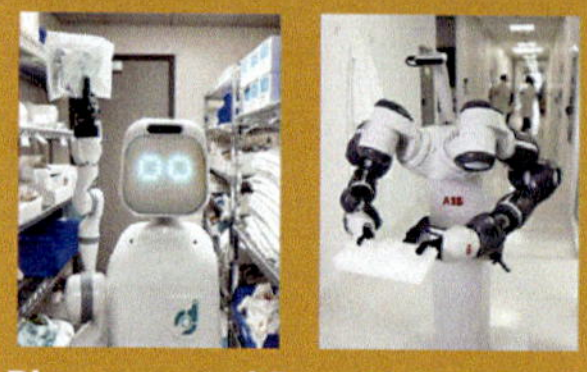

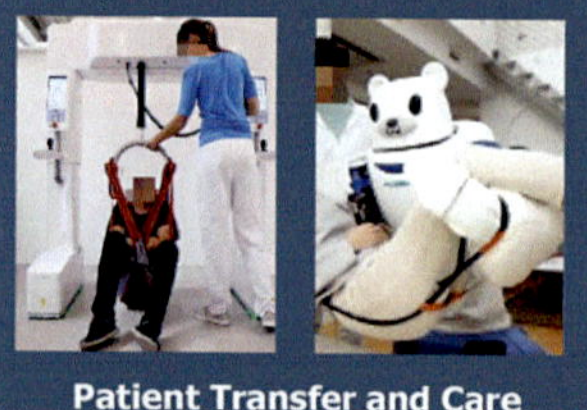

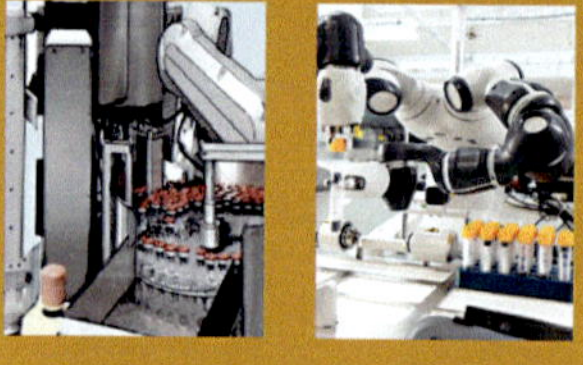

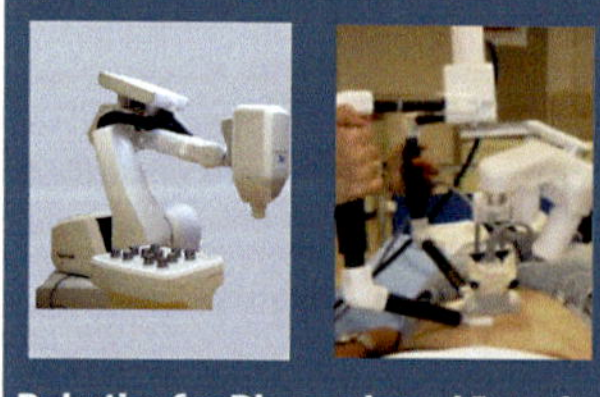

Fig. 6.1 Robotic systems for hospital automation. Robotic systems that are designed for improving the levels of automation in hospitals, which can be categorized into five groups, including robots for hospital logistics (TUG, Aethon © 2018; Guardian II, Guangdong Jaten Robot & Automation Co.,Ltd., © 2022), pharmacy and drug management (YuMi, ABB, © 2023; Moxi, Diligent Robotics Inc., © 2023), patient transfer and care (PTR, copyright by PTR Robots; Robear, copyright by RIKEN, Japan), high-throughput lab automation (Pharma, DSG Robotics, © 2017–2020 by Netech; YuMi, ABB, © 2023), and diagnosis and imaging (CyberKnife, Wikimedia Commons (CC BY 2.0); Melody, adapted from [10], Creative Commons (CC BY 4.0))

work around the clock, leaving human nurses to deal with more high-level tasks that are difficult to automate. With the help of these intelligent robots, the physical demands on human workers can be significantly reduced.

During the COVID-19 pandemic, hospital automation robots were deployed to help reduce exposure to pathogens and ensure a safe environment for both patients and health workers [11, 12]. Robotic systems for high-throughput laboratories can maintain more efficient processes, facilitating research and development of new drugs and therapies [13–16]. Within this field, robots could accelerate the workflow in terms of screening, testing, sequencing, as well as data interpretation and analysis. Robots have also been used for diagnosis and imaging, providing an increasing level of autonomy in hospital care pathways [10, 17].

Although a variety of hospital automation robots have emerged, there is still a lack of systematic approaches for the development and deployment of robotic systems in smart hospitals. In the future, we foresee hospital automation robots working in different scenarios, including clinical care, public safety, laboratory and supply chain automation, and out-of-hospital care, as well as improving the quality of life of patients at homes. These robots could form an ecosystem and improve the capacity and efficiency of future intelligent hospitals.

6.2 Robots for Hospital Logistics

Robots for hospital logistics, as shown in Fig. 6.2, aim to undertake conventional labor-intensive and repetitive tasks like human workers. These robots have demonstrated superiority in efficiency and accuracy compared to their human counterparts.

Every day, clinicians have to spend a lot of time managing the inventory of various warehouses and handling numerous disposable items, medical devices, and medical waste. Another labor-intensive task is in-hospital delivery, where a large number of items are required to be delivered, dispensed, and collected between different places. However, the sequence of these warehouses and wards can be disorganized due to the stressful working environment of a hospital. In addition, disinfection is a significant task in hospitals, which has received increased attention after the outbreak of COVID-19 [11].

To help resolve these issues, various robots for hospital logistics have been developed in the past decades [12–14, 19], with most of them built on mobile platforms. By using visual or LiDAR-based *Simultaneous Localization and Mapping* (SLAM) techniques [20, 21], 2D/3D maps of the environment can be constructed; hence, autonomous mobile robots are able to automatically navigate from one place to another during delivery. To enable reliable navigation in an indoor environment, some emerging technologies, such as Wi-Fi, RFID, or other landmarks, can be utilized to improve the performance of localization [22]. In addition, dynamic object and human detection, object avoidance, and path planning are critical functions of autonomous service robots moving in cluttered hospital environments [23, 24].

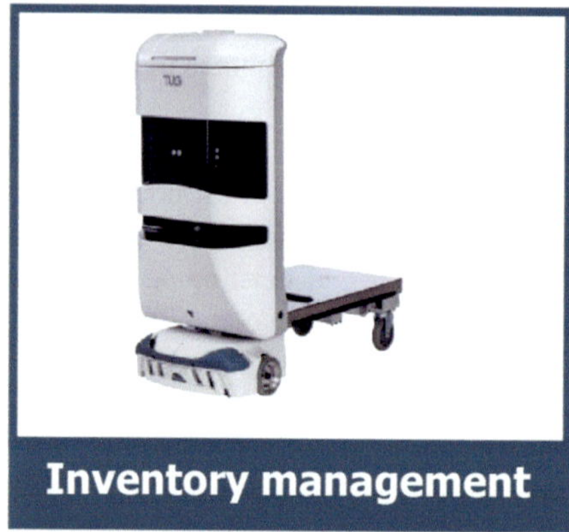

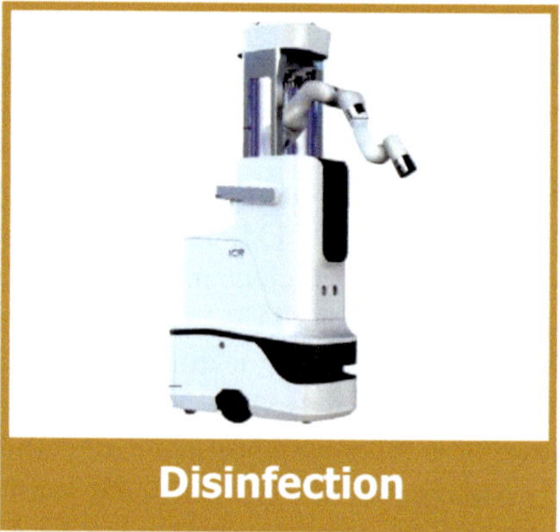

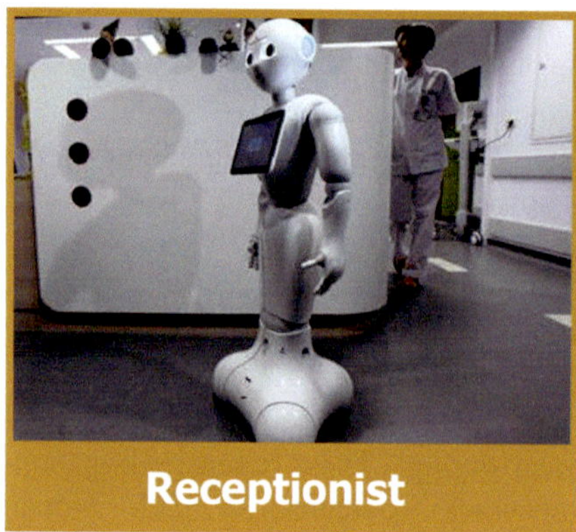

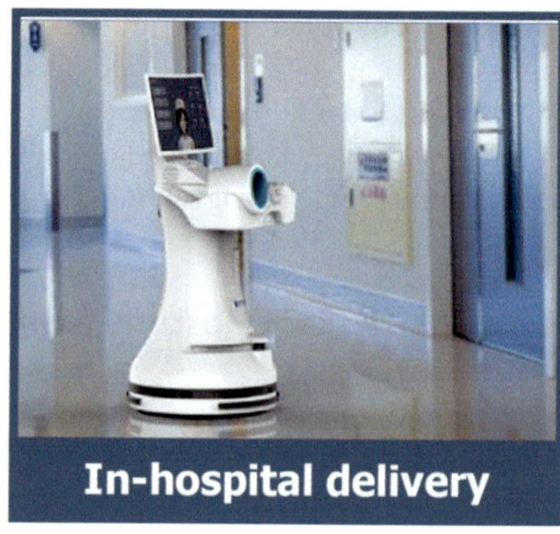

Fig. 6.2 Robots for hospital logistics. The robots can help medical staff with inventory management, disinfection, reception, and in-hospital delivery, such as TUG, Aethon © 2018; Guardian II, Guangdong Jaten Robot & Automation Co.,Ltd., © 2022; Pepper (adapted from [18]); Medical supplies management robot (TMiRob Co. Ltd., © 2017)

Receptionist robots are commonly used to offer guidance about the infrastructures and services of hospitals [25], providing patients with a pleasant experience within hospitals. Commonly, receptionist robots are humanoids, with intelligent speech interaction, where patients can communicate with them directly. This kind of robot is especially attractive in children's hospitals, helping alleviate negative emotions in the course of medical care.

6.3 Robots for Pharmacy and Drug Management

Staff working in the pharmacy department need to pick up and pack thousands of drugs every day, which is tedious and time-consuming. To fulfill the additional requirements in pharmacy management, recent advanced robots are equipped with robotic arms to enable dexterous drug picking and placement, e.g., Moxi (Diligent

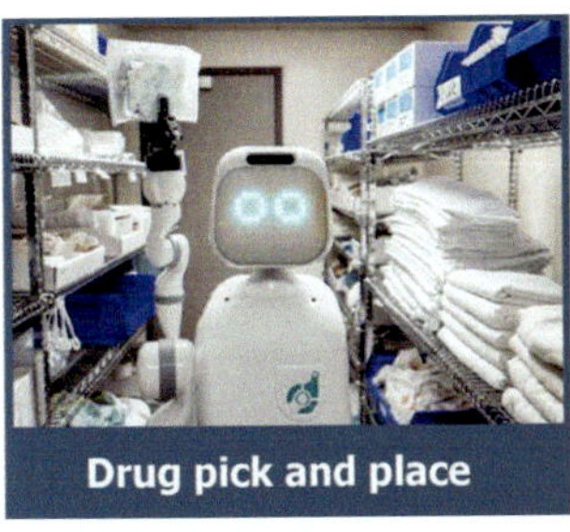

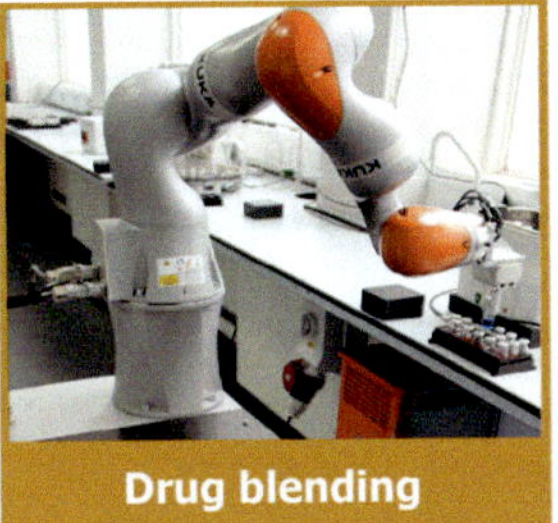

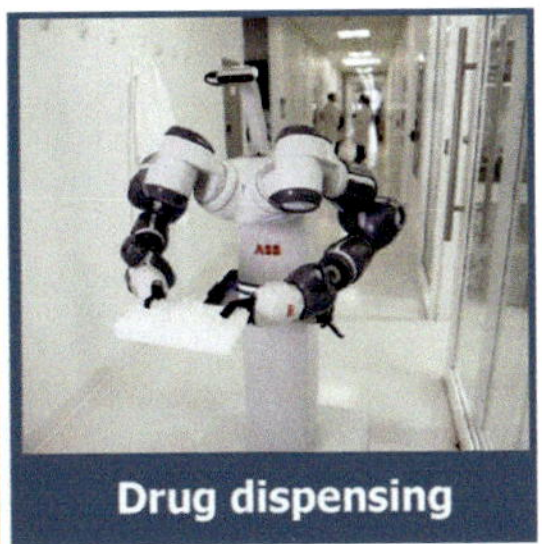

Fig. 6.3 Robots for pharmacy and drug management. From left to right: Moxi (Diligent Robotics Inc., Texas, USA; Diligent Robotics Inc., © 2023); KUKA iiwa (adapted with Springer Nature permission from [26]); YuMi (ABB, Zurich, Switzerland; ABB, © 2023)

Robotics, Texas, USA) and YuMi (ABB, Zurich, Switzerland) robots, as shown in Fig. 6.3. When integrated with advanced computer vision technologies (e.g., object detection, 6D pose estimation) [27], these robots are able to grasp and manipulate different objects like human beings. In addition, through the use of human pose estimation and tracking, they can cooperate with clinicians in a shared workspace. Compared to human workers, robots could provide "zero-error" pharmacy management and avoid potential contamination risks induced by human workers. In addition, for intravenous drugs and anti-tumor drugs, robotic systems can help blend drugs with high speed and throughput.

6.4 Robots for Patient Transfer and Care

In hospitals, patients need to move between different wards or diagnostic departments [28]. For patients with impaired physical functions, frequent transfer from bedside to a wheelchair is difficult. In most cases, the transfer of a patient requires multiple nurses or caregivers. Such a task is one of the most onerous jobs, also representing an occupational risk for nurses or caregivers. Therefore, how to lift and move patients safely and comfortably is of great importance in the design of transfer robots. Furthermore, patient transfer usually occurs in cluttered and unstructured environments, making autonomous robotic manipulation difficult.

In terms of patient transfer, safety is an important prerequisite in robotic system design, and many supporting or fixation mechanisms have been investigated to ensure the safe transport of patients [29]. One of the representative transfer robots is a grounded robotic system, e.g., PTR robots developed by Blue Ocean Robotics. Such a robot is able to transfer patients from bed to wheelchair through the use of an overhanging structure. Another line of research considered the transfer of patients by mimicking human caregivers. As illustrated in the top right of Fig. 6.4, Robear, developed by RIKEN Institute, is equipped with dual robotics arms for supporting and holding disabled patients. In addition, the dual-arm design can help the patient with postural transfer in a more natural way, i.e., sit-to-stand and stand-to-sit. For patients with sufficient motor functions of upper limbs, the transfer robots like UFU

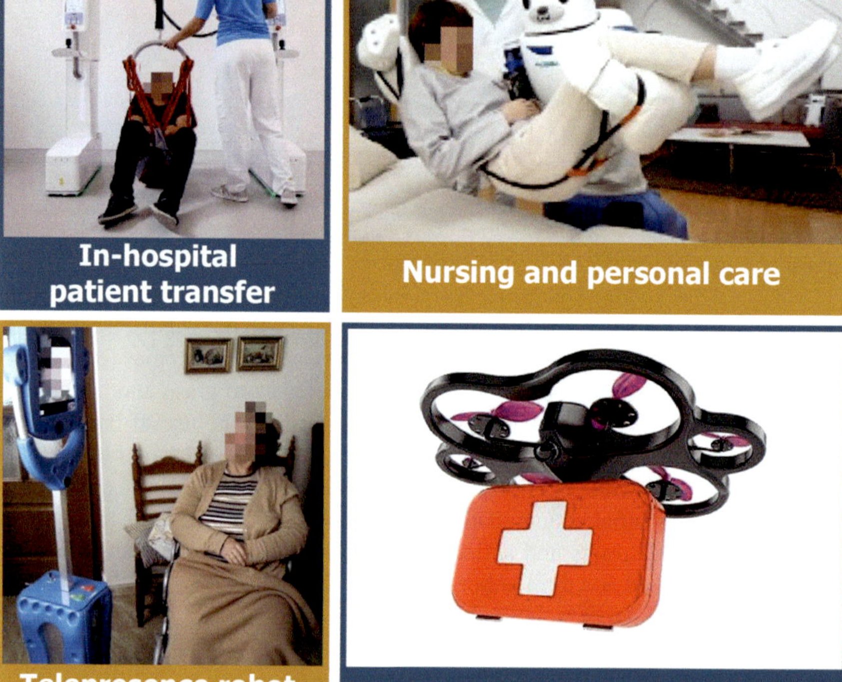

Fig. 6.4 Patient transfer and nursing robots. The robots can provide careful medical service and all-around physical/social care for patients. Top row: PTR robots (Blue Ocean Robotics, Odense, Denmark; Copyright by PTR Robots); Robear (Riken Institute, Japan; Copyright © RIKEN). Bottom row: Giraff (Giraff Technologies AB, Västerås, Sweden; adapted with Springer Nature permission from [30]); UAV (CC BY 4.0)

(RoboCT, Hangzhou, China) aim to support the patients at underarm and shank, allowing a change of posture according to patients' commands [31]. Since the outbreak of COVID-19, a new requirement of inter-hospital or home-to-hospital transfer has been raised [28], i.e., protecting medical staff and patients from potential exposure to risks of infection. However, in the face of a sudden surge in patients with infectious diseases, the limited resources of specialized ambulances cannot meet practical demands. By leveraging recent advances in autonomous driving, robots with dedicated designs to fulfill the requirements of epidemic prevention will potentially solve this problem.

In hospitals, nurses are often overworked due to staff shortages. In future intelligent hospitals, robots can help nurses with simple and repetitive tasks, such as surgical assistance in the operating room, remote inspection rounds, and other tasks.

In the operating rooms, surgical assist nurses are required to prepare surgical tools and assist surgeons during surgery. Although not difficult, these tasks can be repetitive and labor-intensive. Therefore, the development of robotic assistants in the operating room has become a popular topic [32]. Gestonurse, developed by Purdue University, is a system consisting of a robotic arm, which can detect the hand gestures of surgeons and then pick up and pass surgical tools, thus improving the efficiency of workflow in operation rooms.

In wards or intensive care units, nurses are required to frequently check patients' status during the recovery period. In order to alleviate their workload, recent robots are designed to enable automatic ward inspection or teleoperation by clinicians from remote locations [33]. Telepresence robots are able to monitor the status of patients regularly, especially useful for dealing with patients suffering from infectious disease, effectively preventing the clinicians from the potential risk of infection [12]. Moxi robot (Diligent Robotics Inc., Texas, USA) can be used to assist nurses in terms of gathering supplies and delivering them to patients. It can relieve the workload of nurses while maintaining the consistency of the medical care workflow. It is also able to recognize and manipulate objects in order to gather supplies and deliver lab samples.

Delivering immediate first aid to patients after an accident is essential to prevent further trauma. Therefore, ambulance robots are designed to speed up the emergency response and provide care and life support during transport [34]. As demonstrated in the bottom right of Fig. 6.4, *Unmanned Aerial Vehicles* (UAVs) equipped with first aid drugs and *Automated External Defibrillator* (AED) devices can arrive at the emergency location in a short time, providing emergency treatment [35].

6.5 Robots for High-Throughput Lab Automation

High-throughput robotics is an emerging topic in lab automation, which aims to enable high throughput and high efficiency in testing, screening, synthesis, DNA/RNA sequencing, in vitro diagnosis, and data analysis and interpretation. With the help of such robotic systems, the research and development of personalized medicine and novel technologies are accelerating.

Laboratory testing is critical in hospitals, which is a fact that became particularly prominent during the COVID-19 pandemic. The workflow first involves the collection and transportation of specimens and then the delivery to the laboratories for testing. Most specimens are collected from different departments in hospitals, while some are collected outside of hospitals. For screening for COVID-19, a huge number of specimens can be collected and then transported to the laboratory for testing every day. During testing, each step will potentially affect the detection quality and may increase safety issues. In addition, conventional testing consumes a lot of manpower and time in sample handling and data analysis, where accuracy and efficiency cannot be fully guaranteed with such a large workload. To conquer this, robotic systems for testing have emerged to improve the degree of automation in laboratories [36]. Different robotic platforms are used for weighting, drying, cooling, pipetting, and other procedures in the workflow, followed by data storage and analysis. During the COVID-19 pandemic, high-throughput test robots have demonstrated their advantages in efficiency and capacity, while preventing human workers from potential high risks [37].

With the development of molecular biology, functional genomics, proteomics, metabolomics, and single-cell omics, we have entered the era of precision medicine. This offers much potential in diagnosis, prognosis, and therapeutics. In the development of novel drugs, the automated synthesis of lead compounds is the most significant step. In this case, slow manual screening cannot meet the requirements of new drug research and development, as there are numerous novel targets. The emergence of robot-assisted screening technology has greatly shortened the lead time of compound development in drug discovery. By using high-throughput robotic systems, the drug discovery process can be accelerated, and biomedical or cellular events can be repeated and tested in a short time [15, 38]. Burger et al. developed a mobile robotic chemist to automate the procedure for searching improved photocatalysts for hydrogen production from water [26], which achieves six times more activity than the initial formulations.

The importance of proteomics in modern drug research has long been recognized. Proteomics involves the understanding and characterizing of proteins in the categories of structure, function, and interaction. Specifically, sequencing was a laborious, expensive, and personnel-intensive task. Recently, robotics and automation technologies are also affecting the field of proteomics [39–41]. By turning the proteome into data, the proteome in a biological sample is digitized and then interpreted with the help of machine learning or artificial intelligence algorithms to obtain the desired results. Recently, Google released the powerful platform AlphaFold/AlphaFold2 [42], a deep neural network that can generate a highly accurate 3D model of a protein. Robotics facilitates the rapid proteomic assay in proteomic drug screening and clinical research [41].

Cells are the basic units of life. With the emergence of technologies in single-cell isolation, single-cell omics is able to provide unique insights into the understanding of genetics at the cellular level and helps explore the heterogeneity of cells across tissues [43]. The main challenge in single-cell isolation is the integrity, throughput, and sensitivity. In order to achieve the parallel micromanipulation of thousands of cells, automated robotic systems can be used for single-cell isolation through the use of droplets or micromechanical valves [43, 44]. Robotic systems are advantageous in extracting and handling living cells with accuracy, achieving high throughput and high accuracy simultaneously. In addition, as an emerging research field, metabolomics has attracted increasing attention in recent years. High-throughput robots can also contribute to the qualitative and quantitative measurement and analysis of metabolites [45].

In vitro diagnostics involves the diagnosis through human body fluids, cells, and tissues, some of which are the essential sources of clinical diagnostics [46, 47]. This information can provide important references for clinicians to create treatment plans. According to the detection principle, in vitro diagnosis mainly includes biochemical diagnosis, immune diagnosis, molecular diagnosis, microbial diagnosis, clinical diagnosis, and pathological diagnosis. In parallel with the development of micro- and nano-robotics, organ-on-a-chip, referring to a chip to simulate physiological systems of organs, takes the microfluidic chip as the core and integrates different technologies, including cell biology, biological materials, and engineering [48, 49]. These chips can help build a microenvironment in vitro that consists of many living cells and simulates the functional organization interface, biological fluid, and mechanical force. Multiple chips can be used to simulate the absorption, distribution, metabolism, and elimination of drugs in the human body. With the help of robotics and automation, in vitro diagnosis can be highly automated with increased throughput and sensitivity. In addition, robotics systems also enable the flexible customization of the workflow design, speeding up the development of personalized medicine.

6.6 Robots for Diagnosis and Imaging

In the context of hospital automation and clinical care, and on top of the categories previously discussed, robots can also help in facilitating diagnosis and acquisition of medical images. For example, robots can be used to collect biological samples, for PoC diagnosis, in ICU, and also within radiology departments both for diagnosis and for treatment purposes. For a detailed overview of these topics, readers are referred to references [10, 12, 50].

Diagnostic blood testing is a routine clinical procedure that is commonly performed manually. However, the COVID-19 pandemic has highlighted the central role of technologies in responding to infectious diseases by protecting medical staff from the risk of infection [12]. Robot-assisted blood testing is one example. HaemoBot and VenousPro are robotic systems that rely on ultrasound guidance and force sensing to automatically locate the vein on a person's forearm and perform cannulation [12]. More recently, researchers at the Italian Institute of Technology have developed a handheld robot for peripheral venous catheterization for pediatric applications [51]. For the diagnosis of infectious diseases, oropharyngeal and nasopharyngeal swabbing is widely used. This requires sample collection, handling, transfer, and laboratory testing. However, the number of qualified medical staff for this process may be limited, as demonstrated by the recent COVID-19 emergency. In such a situation, the deployment of autonomous robots for nasopharyngeal and oropharyngeal swabbing can be extremely helpful and safer, as the medical staff do not need to be in close contact with the person to be tested. A low-cost robot that can be remotely controlled has been developed for collecting nasopharyngeal specimens. The system includes an active end-effector, a passive robot arm for positioning, and a detachable swab gripper with integrated force sensing [52].

Telerobotics—by combining human operator knowledge and a remotely controlled robot—can be helpful in applications where a remote doctor takes all the physiological parameters and diagnoses a disease using audiovisual aids [50]. Exemplary applications are telepresence robots for POC diagnosis and for ICU patients [12]. POC robots can be used for patient–doctor teleconsultations and to perform physical examinations such as auscultation and palpation [53]. POC robots can provide rapid test results to patients, supporting on-the-spot clinical decision-making, and can combine portable imaging or sensing devices with integrated hospital information systems [12]. ICU robots can be used to provide access to off-site patients, supervising physicians, and other specialists, making otherwise very difficult procedures possible [12].

In 2005, the UCLA Medical Center used an RP-6 robot (InTouch Health, Santa Barbara, USA) in its neurosurgery ICUs. It was controlled by a webcam and joystick over a broad-band connection [54]. iRobot and InTouch Health announced an alliance targeting healthcare in 2011, and the Remote Presence Virtual + Independent Telemedicine Assistant (RP-VITA) robot was unveiled in 2012. In 2013, the FDA cleared RP-VITA as the first autonomously navigating telepresence robot in healthcare [55]. RP-VITA has remote interactive capability between clinicians and patients. It has enhanced navigation capabilities (based on environment mapping and obstacle avoidance tailored to hospital environments), and it offers virtual assessment and monitoring of patients and provides virtual visits for the family members of patients.

In addition to telepresence and telemedicine (we do not include surgical robots here as already discussed in Chap. 3), robots can be employed for the remote acquisition of medical images and robot-assisted therapies. For example, robotic ultrasound is the fusion of a robotic system and an ultrasound station with its probe attached to the robot end-effector. This combination might overcome ultrasound disadvantages by means of either a teleoperated, a collaborative assisting, or even an autonomous system [10]. Using a robot to perform ultrasound imaging poses task-specific challenges, such as position, access window, and force control of the robotic arm in order to obtain reliable images while maintaining a safe procedure. The commercially available robotic arm UR5 (Universal Robots) has been used to develop a general, low-cost robotic ultrasound platform that integrates haptic control [56]. A 5G-based robot-assisted remote ultrasound system for cardiopulmonary assessment of patients with COVID-19 has been investigated by Chai et al. [57] Commercially available ultrasound robots include the MGIUS-R3 (MGI Tech Co.) system and the MELODY (AdEchoTech) system. MGIUS-R3 consists of a 6-DoF robotic arm, including a force sensor and an ultrasound probe, which is remotely controlled. A feasibility study was conducted to assess the remote examination of a patient with COVID-19 [58]. MELODY is a robotic probe holder at the patient site. The coarse positioning of the robot is handled by a clinical assistant, while fine adjustments of probe orientation are remotely controlled by the expert sonographer via a haptic device with force feedback. Applications of MELODY include cardiac, abdominal, obstetric, pelvic, and vascular telesonography [59] in over 300 patients. A detailed review of ultrasound robots is reported by von Haxthausen et al. [10]

Robotic systems are also utilized in radiology to reduce the level of radiation and safety issues for human operators. The Multitom Rax (Siemens Healthineers, Erlangen, Germany) offers fluoroscopy, angiography, and 3D imaging to perform a multitude of X-rays in one room where the physician can see 3D images in real time as the robot moves around the patient. Artis Zeego (Siemens Healthineers, Erlangen,

Germany) and Discovery (GE Healthcare, Chicago, USA) are commercially available robotic systems that allow image guidance during interventional angiography. Both systems can operate as real-time 2D fluoroscopy and as rapid 3D fluoroscopy CT-like imaging systems, providing uninterrupted, unobstructed access to the surgical area and full flexibility to patient positioning. The Discovery system provides advanced image guidance for endovascular procedures, enabling 3D image fusion and navigation through advanced software solutions (i.e., ASSIST software) for aneurysm repairs and aortic valve replacement [3].

CyberKnife (Accuray Inc., Sunnyvale, CA) is a commercially available robot for radiotherapy of cancer patients. It is a minimally invasive robotic system that delivers stereotactic radiosurgery and stereotactic body radiation therapy treatments anywhere in the body (e.g., cranial and spinal tumors, prostate, lung, liver, and pancreas cancers) with high-tech robotic precision and integrated real-time motion synchronization. CyberKnife contains integrated imaging systems that can automatically detect and compensate for motion, allowing for frameless treatment. Throughout treatment, the radiosurgical target is continually sensed using a combination of X-ray and optical imaging. The target pose is localized into a common reference frame using a combination of image registration algorithms and precisely calibrated coordinate transformations. CyberKnife tracks and autonomously adapts to tumor or patient movement during treatment to deliver a maximum dose of radiation directly to the tumor while preserving healthy organs and tissues. For organs that move with respiration, CyberKnife synchronizes its motion to the target anatomy on the basis of a learned model and multimodal sensing [3]. A technical overview of the CyberKnife system is presented by Kilby et al. [60]

6.7 Conclusions

With increasing needs for high-standard medical services, an emerging area in medical robotics is to develop robotics systems for hospital automation. These robots are designed to either help reduce the workload of medical staff or facilitate tedious examination or testing procedures. In this chapter, we have outlined existing hospital automation robots and categorized them into five groups according to their functionalities: hospital logistics, pharmacy and drug management, patient transfer and care, high-throughput lab automation, and diagnosis and imaging. For each subcategory, the main research focus and available systems were discussed. In the next chapter, we will outline new opportunities and emerging technologies for medical robotics in general.

References

1. Gentili A. Answering the great automation question. Sci Robot. 2022;7(65):eabo7210.
2. Yang G-Z, Bellingham J, Dupont PE, et al. The grand challenges of science robotics. Sci Robot. 2018;3(14):eaar7650.

3. Troccaz J, Dagnino G, Yang G-Z. Frontiers of medical robotics: from concept to systems to clinical translation. Annu Rev Biomed Eng. 2019;21:193–218.
4. Vitiello V, Lee S-L, Cundy TP, et al. Emerging robotic platforms for minimally invasive surgery. IEEE Rev Biomed Eng. 2012;6:111–26.
5. Tejima N. Rehabilitation robotics: a review. Adv Robot. 2001;14(7):551–64.
6. Chang WH, Kim YH. Robot-assisted therapy in stroke rehabilitation. J Stroke. 2013;15(3):174–81.
7. Jouaiti M, Henaff P. Robot-based motor rehabilitation in autism: a systematic review. Int J Soc Robot. 2019;11(5):753–64.
8. Breazeal C, Dautenhahn K, Kanda T. Social robotics. In: Siciliano B, Khatib O, editors. Springer handbook of robotics. Cham: Springer; 2016. p. 1935–72.
9. Linge S. Robots in hospitals: how could a robot in a hospital look like? 2019. https://www.diva-portal.org/smash/record.jsf?pid=diva2%3A1330132&dswid=8671.
10. von Haxthausen F, Böttger S, Wulff D, et al. Medical robotics for ultrasound imaging: current systems and future trends. Curr Robot Rep. 2021;2(1):55–71.
11. Yang G-ZJ, Nelson B, Murphy RR, et al. Combating COVID-19—the role of robotics in managing public health and infectious diseases. Am Assoc Adv Sci. 2020;5:eabb5589.
12. Gao A, Murphy RR, Chen W, et al. Progress in robotics for combating infectious diseases. Sci Robot. 2021;6(52):eabf1462.
13. Bloss R. Mobile hospital robots cure numerous logistic needs. Ind Robot. 2011;38(6):567–71.
14. Rodriguez-Gonzalez CG, Herranz-Alonso A, Escudero-Vilaplana V, et al. Robotic dispensing improves patient safety, inventory management, and staff satisfaction in an outpatient hospital pharmacy. J Eval Clin Pract. 2019;25(1):28–35.
15. Macarron R, Banks MN, Bojanic D, et al. Impact of high-throughput screening in biomedical research. Nat Rev Drug Discov. 2011;10(3):188–95.
16. Gu E, Tang X, Langner S, et al. Robot-based high-throughput screening of antisolvents for lead halide perovskites. Joule. 2020;4(8):1806–22.
17. Subramanian V, Ragunath K. Advanced endoscopic imaging: a review of commercially available technologies. Clin Gastroenterol Hepatol. 2014;12(3):368–76.e1.
18. France-presse. https://www.theguardian.com/technology/2016/jun/14/robot-receptionists-hospitals-belgium-pepper-humanoid.
19. Guettari M, Gharbi I, Hamza S. UVC disinfection robot. Environ Sci Pollut Res. 2021;28(30):40394–9.
20. Hess W, Kohler D, Rapp H, et al. Real-time loop closure in 2D LIDAR SLAM. In: Proceedings of the 2016 IEEE international conference on robotics and automation (ICRA). IEEE; 2016.
21. Mur-Artal R, Tardós JD. ORB-SLAM2: an open-source slam system for monocular, stereo, and RGB-D cameras. IEEE Trans Robot. 2017;33(5):1255–62.
22. Chen Z, Zou H, Jiang H, et al. Fusion of WiFi, smartphone sensors and landmarks using the Kalman filter for indoor localization. Sensors. 2015;15(1):715–32.
23. Yazdi M, Bouwmans T. New trends on moving object detection in video images captured by a moving camera: a survey. Comput Sci Rev. 2018;28:157–77.
24. Zhang H-Y, Lin W-M, Chen A-X. Path planning for the mobile robot: a review. Symmetry. 2018;10(10):450.
25. Karabegović I, Doleček V. The role of service robots and robotic systems in the treatment of patients in medical institutions. Adv Technol Syst Appl. 2017:9–25.
26. Burger B, Maffettone PM, Gusev VV, et al. A mobile robotic chemist. Nature. 2020;583(7815):237–41.
27. Billard A, Kragic D. Trends and challenges in robot manipulation. Science. 2019;364(6446):eaat8414.
28. Kulshrestha A, Singh J. Inter-hospital and intra-hospital patient transfer: recent concepts. Indian J Anaesth. 2016;60(7):451.
29. Huang Z, Lin C, Kanai-Pak M, et al. Robot patient design to simulate various patients for transfer training. IEEE/ASME Trans Mechatron. 2017;22(5):2079–90.

30. González-Jiménez J, Galindo C, Ruiz-Sarmiento J Technical improvements of the Giraff telepresence robot based on users' evaluation. In: Proceedings of the 2012 IEEE RO-MAN: the 21st IEEE international symposium on robot and human interactive communication. IEEE; 2012.
31. Wu R, Wang J, Chen W, et al. Design of a transfer robot for the assistance of elderly and disabled. Adv Robot. 2021;35(3–4):194–204.
32. Jacob M, Li Y-T, Akingba G, et al. Gestonurse: a robotic surgical nurse for handling surgical instruments in the operating room. J Robot Surg. 2012;6(1):53–63.
33. Haque A, Milstein A, Fei-Fei L. Illuminating the dark spaces of healthcare with ambient intelligence. Nature. 2020;585(7824):193–202.
34. Samani H, Zhu R. Robotic automated external defibrillator ambulance for emergency medical service in smart cities. IEEE Access. 2016;4:268–83.
35. Scudellari M. Drone beats ambulance in race to deliver first aid to patients. IEEE Spectrum. https://spectrum.ieee.org/the-human-os/biomedical/devices/drone-vs-ambulance-drone-wins. Accessed 20 Mar 2020.
36. Chapman T. Lab automation and robotics: automation on the move. Nature. 2003;421(6923):661–3.
37. Shental N, Levy S, Wuvshet V, et al. Efficient high-throughput SARS-CoV-2 testing to detect asymptomatic carriers. Sci Adv. 2020;6(37):eabc5961.
38. Greenaway R, Santolini V, Bennison M, et al. High-throughput discovery of organic cages and catenanes using computational screening fused with robotic synthesis. Nat Commun. 2018;9(1):1–11.
39. Lesley SA. High-throughput proteomics: protein expression and purification in the postgenomic world. Protein Expr Purif. 2001;22(2):159–64.
40. Alterovitz G, Liu J, Chow J, et al. Automation, parallelism, and robotics for proteomics. Proteomics. 2006;6(14):4016–22.
41. Messner CB, Demichev V, Bloomfield N, et al. Ultra-fast proteomics with scanning SWATH. Nat Biotechnol. 2021;39(7):846–54.
42. Jumper J, Evans R, Pritzel A, et al. Highly accurate protein structure prediction with AlphaFold. Nature. 2021;596(7873):583–9.
43. Fazal S, Azam S. Robotics in single-cell omics. In: Barh D, Azevedo V, editors. Single cell omics. Oxford: Elsevier; 2019. p. 381–95.
44. Ungai-Salánki R, Gerecsei T, Fürjes P, et al. Automated single cell isolation from suspension with computer vision. Sci Rep. 2016;6(1):1–9.
45. Zampieri M, Sekar K, Zamboni N, et al. Frontiers of high-throughput metabolomics. Curr Opin Chem Biol. 2017;36:15–23.
46. Zhou W, Gao X, Liu D, et al. Gold nanoparticles for in vitro diagnostics. Chem Rev. 2015;115(19):10575–636.
47. Sun X, Wan JJ, Qian K. Designed microdevices for in vitro diagnostics. Small Methods. 2017;1(10):1700196.
48. Zhang B, Korolj A, Lai BFL, et al. Advances in organ-on-a-chip engineering. Nat Rev Mater. 2018;3(8):257–78.
49. Wu Q, Liu J, Wang X, et al. Organ-on-a-chip: recent breakthroughs and future prospects. Biomed Eng Online. 2020;19(1):1–19.
50. Khan ZH, Siddique A, Lee CW. Robotics utilization for healthcare digitization in global COVID-19 management. Int J Environ Res Public Health. 2020;17(11):3819.
51. Cheng Z, Davies BL, Caldwell DG, et al. A hand-held robot for precise and safe PIVC. IEEE Robot Automat Lett. 2019;4(2):655–61.
52. Wang S, Wang K, Tang R, et al. Design of a low-cost miniature robot to assist the COVID-19 nasopharyngeal swab sampling. IEEE Trans Med Robot Bion. 2020;3(1):289–93.
53. Yang G, Lv H, Zhang Z, et al. Keep healthcare workers safe: application of teleoperated robot in isolation ward for COVID-19 prevention and control. Chinese J Mech Eng. 2020;33(1):1–4.
54. Becevic M, Clarke MA, Alnijoumi MM, et al. Robotic telepresence in a medical intensive care unit—clinicians' perceptions. Perspect Health Inf Manag. 2015;12(Summer):1c.

55. Ackerman E. Telepresence robots are helping take pressure off hospital staff. IEEE Spectrum: Technology, Engineering, and Science News. 2020.
56. Mathiassen K, Fjellin JE, Glette K, et al. An ultrasound robotic system using the commercial robot UR5. Front Robot AI. 2016;3:1.
57. Chai H-H, Ye R-Z, Xiong L-F, et al. Successful use of a 5G-based robot-assisted remote ultrasound system in a care center for disabled patients in rural China. Front Public Health. 2022;10
58. Wang J, Peng C, Zhao Y, et al. Application of a robotic tele-echography system for COVID-19 pneumonia. J Ultrasound Med. 2021;40(2):385–90.
59. Adams SJ, Burbridge BE, Badea A, et al. A crossover comparison of standard and telerobotic approaches to prenatal sonography. J Ultrasound Med. 2018;37(11):2603–12.
60. Kilby W, Naylor M, Dooley JR, et al. A technical overview of the CyberKnife system. In: Nasab MHA, editor. Handbook of robotic and image-guided surgery. Oxford: Elsevier; 2020. p. 15–38.

Emerging Challenges and Future Trends 7

Contents

The prosperity of robotics, mechanical engineering, material science, artificial intelligence, and biomedical engineering has an increasing impact on the conventional medical industry [1–3]. With the close integration of medicine and engineering, medical robotics has emerged for automated diagnosis, treatment, rehabilitation, and disease management, providing high-quality medical services for the general population.

Advances in relevant technologies and increasing demand from people for high-quality medical services are driving the rapid uptake of medical robotics. The aging population has led to an increasing incidence of malignant tumors, cardiovascular and cerebrovascular diseases, and neurological disorders. However, limited medical resources cannot fully meet the requirements of such a huge rise in medical expenses. Medical robots can assist clinicians in completing accurate disease diagnosis and treatment [4–9], improving the quality of medical services. In addition, robot-assisted rehabilitation training can greatly shorten postoperative rehabilitation and accelerate the recovery of patients who have survived severe diseases, such as stroke [10–14]. Personal assistance of the elderly and disabled people has also

Y. Guo et al., *Medical Robotics*, Innovative Medical Devices,
https://doi.org/10.1007/978-981-99-7317-0_7

become an important responsibility of society, leading to a huge demand for assistive robots in daily life, reducing the requirements for professional nurses or caregivers [15–19]. In addition, medical robots have demonstrated their capabilities in improving the automation levels of hospitals, ranging from hospital service to high throughput testing and screening [20–23].

7.1 Commercial and Investment Trends

In recent years, the global market of medical robotics has grown rapidly, with a *Compound Annual Growth Rate* (CAGR) of around 15%. The total size was expected to reach $20.7 billion by 2021, as shown in Fig. 7.1. Among three categories of medical robotics, the market size of surgical robotics is the largest (around 46%), and the growth rate of rehabilitation and assistive robot is the fastest.

According to the Industry *Analysis Research Consulting* (ARC) Analysis released in 2014, North America occupies around 40% of the total global market for medical robotics, and Europe accounts for 32% of the market. It can be seen from Fig. 7.2 that European and American enterprises are currently in a dominant position in the global medical robotics market. Intuitive Surgical Inc., established in 1995, is the leading company in surgical robotics, where its market value exceeded $1000 billion in 2021. After FDA approval in 2000, there are around 7000 da Vinci surgical robot systems launched worldwide. In addition to North America and Europe, Asia-Pacific is an emerging area with rapid growth in medical robotics research and development, in which a number of startups have been established recently.

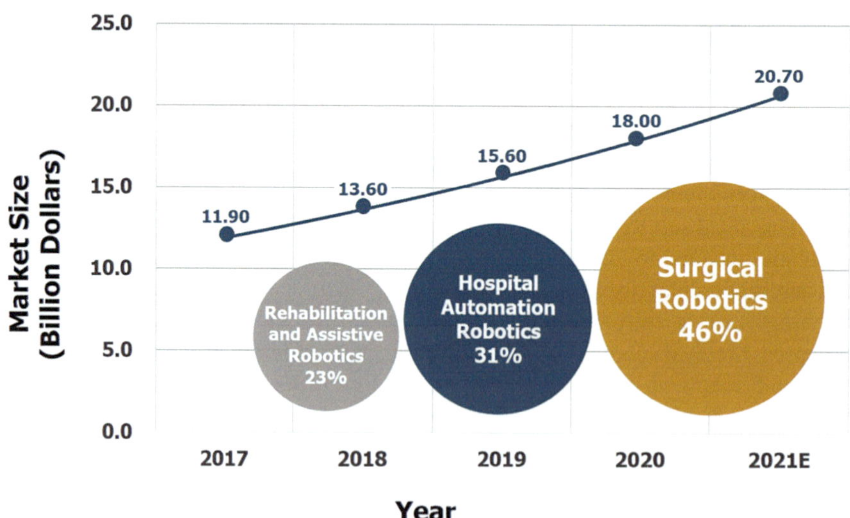

Fig. 7.1 Market size of medical robotics in recent 5 years

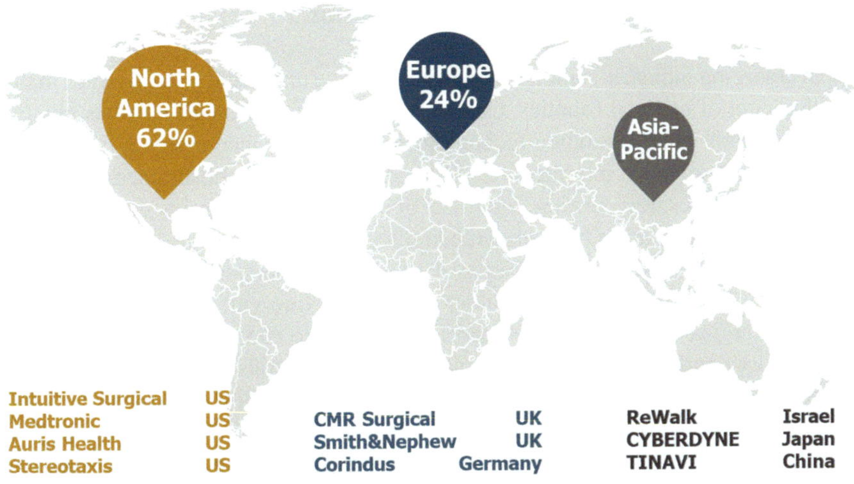

Fig. 7.2 The distribution of the global market of medical robotics

7.2 Ethics, Regulations, and Legal Considerations

7.2.1 Ethics

Medical robots are set to impact many aspects of our lives, which can inevitably raise new ethical and safety issues [24]. Considering there will be numerous medical robots with high levels of automation in the future, clinicians may heavily rely on these intelligent systems and gradually lose some skills. When mistakes happen, clinicians may have less responsibility due to the high level of control and supervision delegated to robots [24].

In addition, medical robots need to collect different kinds of data directly from patients to enable accurate diagnosis, treatment, and personal assistance. Particularly for rehabilitation and assistive robots, diverse human–machine interfaces will record the real-time physiological signals of human subjects, such as EEG, EMG, gaze, and heart rate. Moreover, video monitoring has been frequently used in different robotic systems for analyzing the movement and cognition behaviors of patients. Hence, data privacy and data protection have become urgent issues, not only in commercial products but also in research and development.

Thanks to the recent advances in deep learning and artificial intelligence, medical robotics systems are integrated with diverse learning-based algorithms to achieve complicated tasks in unstructured environments. Hence, another typical ethical issue exists in most artificial intelligence algorithms as they may be trained with limited data with biased distributions, noisy labels, or incomplete observations. With respect to these models, medical robots may overlook the differences between patients, such as customs, cultural beliefs, and gender, leading to potential prejudice and discrimination in decision-making.

7.2.2 Regulations and Legal Considerations

As an emerging industry, standardization has become one of the critical issues in the development of medical robotics. Currently, most available medical robots involve different kinds of open-source technologies, leading to inconsistency across the hardware and software interfaces. It is also desirable to establish a series of standards in terms of safety, testing, interface, or even core components of robots, thus facilitating the adaptation from research to relevant industries. As medical products, medical robots are facing very strict assessment and supervision. The fact is that it may take a long time to get regulatory approval before entering the market. For instance, surgical robots typically need several years to complete sufficient clinical trials before approval. On the other hand, different countries have their own certification and regulation systems [e.g., FDA in the USA, CE in Europe, *National Medical Products Administration* (NMPA) in China], which may add further hurdles for medical robots entering the global market. To alleviate this difficulty, some regions have opened a green certification channel for accelerated clinical use of some innovative and safe medical robot products.

In addition to aforementioned ethic issues, regulatory and legal considerations need to be addressed, especially for clarifying clear responsibilities of clinicians, robots, and companies. First, regulations and laws should indicate responsible access to data, including users, clinicians, technicians, developers, and overseers from the government. In addition, data encryption and storage need careful consideration to ensure privacy and safety. More importantly, there should be a worldwide association to develop relevant international standards.

7.3 Opportunities and Challenges of Surgical Robotics

Increasing technological advances as well as clinical demands—especially in the last decade—have propelled the development of surgical robotics. As analyzed in Chaps. 2 and 3, the scientific community has addressed a multitude of surgical challenges by proposing new robotic devices and introducing novel clinical methodologies and workflows. Recent work in the field of surgical robotics focuses on miniaturizing and increasing the level of autonomy of new surgical platforms, making robotic systems smaller, smarter, and more versatile. Remarkably, many new technologies are closely linked to endoluminal interventions, underpinning the importance of such procedures for research activities in the next decade. In the following paragraphs, we outline some potential opportunities and challenges for surgical robotics that the scientific and clinical communities are expected to face in the coming years.

7.3.1 Improving User Experience

Various effective and efficient HMIs are the essential components of forming HRI in robotic surgery and will present a key element for next-generation devices to achieve acceptance among clinical operators. Novel HRI is expected to provide clinicians with intuitive and transparent control of surgical robots, enabling a higher level of cooperation and transition to manual workflows at any time and effectively communicating procedural phases and AI-driven decision support.

In the last decade, various HRI concepts have been proposed. Most of the commercial and academic platforms still use conventional joysticks that are mapped to the robot end-effector to perform the desired task, e.g., instrument displacement, feeding, rotation, and bending. However, the use of a conventional joystick is often counterintuitive for clinical users, as it does not allow the capture of surgical skills that have been acquired over years of training and experience.

This limitation has been addressed in research through different strategies, such as designing task-specific HRI or abstracting the input layer to novel concepts and feedback cues. An example is the tailored HRI for endovascular surgery created at Imperial College London (see Chap. 3 and the research by Kundrat et al. [8]) that mimics the clinical handling and motion pattern of conventional catheters and guidewires. Similarly, flexible electronic circuits are proposed for the implementation of customized HRI to enhance user control and feedback of soft robots in endoscopy [25]. Alternative strategies include mapping the device input to high-level interfaces supported by visual or haptic cues. Recent work in bronchoscopy proposed gesture-based robot control or AR-based planning and monitoring of surgical intervention [26]. This enables interactive definition and execution of robotic motion as well as an overlay of procedural data.

7.3.2 Surgical Vision and Navigation Inside the Human Body

Accurate navigation of luminal organs is of exceptional importance for precision surgery and safety [27]. To date, the clinical operator predominantly navigates the device (whether robotic or not) based on anatomical knowledge, experience, and vision provided by the embedded imaging system. The evolution of imaging and sensing has driven the development of navigation frameworks [28]. This is not limited to external sensing or integration of fiber-optics to the endoluminal hardware [e.g., Ion Endoluminal System (Intuitive Surgical, Sunnyvale, USA)] to capture the shape or pose of the surgical instrument with respect to the human anatomy, but also includes tracking of devices and tissue in the field of view as well as view expansion. Although emerging technologies have been studied in preclinical and clinical settings, their application in clinical routines remains challenging due to individual procedural requirements. Future work is dedicated to the identification of clinical tasks that benefit from novel technologies, e.g., less time needed to navigate the endoluminal device to a certain pathological tissue and improved lesion detection from functional imaging.

Major technological leaps are achieved by emerging endoscopic imaging modalities [29]. White-light imaging of the luminal environment using fiber-based or chip-on-tip sensors is still the gold standard in clinical routine and pathology assessment. This also applies to vision-based robot control frameworks. Enhanced sensitivity is presented by multimodal imaging, e.g., a combination of *Narrow-Band Imaging* (NBI) or hyperspectral imaging and white-light imaging, which has already entered clinical routines in gastrointestinal procedures and facilitates the detection of lesions [30]. The next generation of imaging is already led by biophotonics that can be integrated into robotic endoscopes and may enable—after functional imaging and in situ diagnostics—a robotic treatment of detected pathologies [31].

7.3.3 Increasing Autonomy in Robotic Surgery

Surgical robotic platforms provide clinicians with superhuman dexterity, superior imaging, and novel opportunities for minimally invasive interventions. However, as we have seen in Chap. 3, the majority of current systems are teleoperated, i.e., taking direct input mapping from clinical operators. Currently, this is the gold standard in robotic surgery and reflects the lowest autonomy level according to the taxonomy presented by Yang et al. [24], with six independent autonomy levels in total (see Fig. 7.3 and Sect. 3.3.1). This definition comprises no autonomy (lowest level) with robotic control based on direct operator input to fully autonomous execution and completion of the robotic task without human interaction (highest level).

Currently, only partial autonomy of workflow phases, i.e., fully predictable device behaviors, are realized in commercial devices. For example, the sequences of motion primitives are executed automatically to support teleoperation. Laparoscopic surgical robots have proven successful under continuous operator control and so currently offer only limited robotic assistance. Orthopedic robots are capable of autonomously milling out a prescribed cavity for knee and hip implants. Endovascular robots are examples of clinical applications for which robotic solutions have yet to be developed, although they could potentially benefit from robotic solutions [1].

Driven by advances in AI [32], fundamental research efforts in endoluminal robotics target increased autonomy levels to support clinical operators and to realize even better clinical outcomes [33]. Autonomous cannulation of targets in the vasculature represents a highly relevant clinical use case [34]. The integration of robotics, computer assistance, and control enables autonomous manipulation and navigation of magnetic endoscopes. Partial autonomy enables cooperation between the surgeon and the robot in certain situations, e.g., navigating challenging anatomy. However, there is a lack of clinical studies involving autonomous behavior with the exception of robotic laparoscopic surgery [9, 32]. Recently, autonomous robotic anastomosis of the intestine has been performed in vivo on porcine models using a setup of two robotic arms with a suturing device and endoscopic vision [35].

Despite ongoing efforts toward robot autonomy in surgery, progress is still incremental. One considerable challenge is the hesitancy and gradual acceptance of

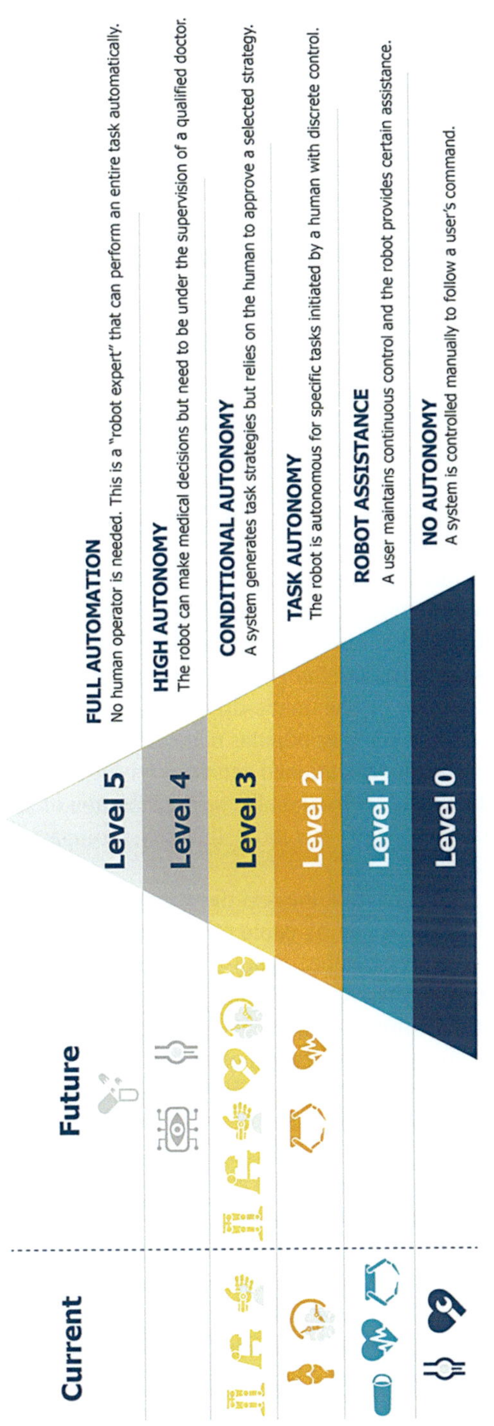

Fig. 7.3 Current and future automation levels of several representative medical robots

robotic devices for surgical applications. On top of this, increasing the level of autonomy of surgical robots significantly impacts the regulatory processes. These must consider—as mentioned above—ethical and safety aspects, as well as further demands for novel concepts to communicate the benefits of autonomy to both users and patients. This is a key factor in clinical translation, acceptance, and usability of the next generation of surgical robotics systems.

7.4 Opportunities and Challenges of Rehabilitation and Assistive Robotics

7.4.1 Soft Materials for Actuation

Compared to conventional geared motors, direct-drive technology combined with a compliant control strategy promotes the miniaturization of motors to provide sufficient driving force on the actuated joints. Series elastic actuators, frequently employed in prosthetics, output the force that is proportional to the position difference multiplied by their spring constant.

Soft materials have demonstrated great potential in developing lightweight actuators, especially for wearable robotic systems. Pneumatic-driven actuators have emerged in rehabilitation and assistive robotics recently, which is advantageous in generating the uniform forces required. Origami-based structure designs have thus far been explored in the development of pneumatic-driven rehabilitation and assistive robotics. Shape memory alloy is another popular material that can be used for designing actuators. Currently, the aforementioned actuators have their own limitations; hence, research attention will be focused on the next generation of soft actuators. These are expected to have high accuracy, linearity, compactness, and driving force.

On the other hand, recent studies have witnessed the successful applications of soft materials in wearable exosuits. Driven by cable or pneumatic actuators, these systems have shown comparative performance against rigid ones. In addition, the cable-driven structure can be well deployed in human suits, enabling power augmentation in a simple manner. Additionally, materials with variable stiffness were explored in the robotic systems for personal assistance. Specifically, strength, flexibility, and fabrication are the key challenges in the next generation of soft wearable robotics for rehabilitation and personal assistance.

7.4.2 Human-Centered and Explainable AI

Intelligent rehabilitation and assistive robotic systems are expected to interact and collaborate with humans to achieve the same task through the detection of human intention, with the aim of compensating or enhancing human capabilities. During rehabilitation training and personal assistance, humans and robots need to establish a mutual understanding of each other's capabilities and respective roles. Therefore, the development of human-centered AI algorithms for enabling human-in-the-loop learning and inference is still an open challenge [36].

Although human intention detection has been successfully incorporated into rehabilitation and assistive robotics, previous works mainly focused on people with physical impairment. Results have shown that it is still challenging to distinguish fine-grade motor intent, such as the movement of an individual finger. Recent achievements in implantable neural interfaces have shown their capability in collecting high-quality brain/neuron activities, facilitating a more accurate and real-time intention detection of fine-grained movements. Furthermore, the research effort should be focused on the detection of high-level cognitive status (e.g., attitude, attention, engagement, emotion, etc.), especially during intervention on patients with cognitive impairments. Such information could be implied in human voice, body language, gaze, head pose, and facial micro-expression.

Social robots provide rehabilitation and intervention for patients with neurological disorders, such as ASD and dementia. Patients exhibit their behavioral and cognitive characteristics in an atypical and unusual way, leading to significant challenges in understanding social activities. Therefore, to tackle the heterogeneity of human subjects, the development of personalized machine learning or deep learning algorithms has attracted extensive attention [37]. Furthermore, users need to understand how interactions with robots are driven, which is a perquisite for establishing the trust of human users, and thus motivating the development of explainable AI [38]. Medical robotic systems are expected to provide understandable explanations to clinicians and patients at the end of a learning or reasoning task.

7.4.3 Social Robotics and Embodied AI

Currently, most existing rehabilitation and assistive robots focus on patients with physical impairment. With an increasing number of patients suffering from neurological disorders, there is a pressing need for robots in cognitive rehabilitation and assistance. Specifically, social robots empowered by embodied AI are expected to act as human therapists. They are expected to effectively interact with the environment and human targets and perform appropriate behavior based on the meaningful interpretation of multimodal perceptual data, thus achieving continuous evolvement in learning, understanding, and social interaction capabilities.

To achieve this goal, social robots need to make decisions through the analysis of data on multiple temporal scales, involving perception, hierarchical information extraction and memorization, and life-long learning paradigms and adaptation [39]. Although recent deep models have achieved promising results, they are computationally expensive and require a huge amount of data for training, which may impede their applications in mobile robotics scenarios and their generalization capability in novel tasks. In addition, the embedded algorithms have to deal with noise, variability, and uncertainty existing in data.

At the system level, integrating the perceptual and computational modules into the robotics system with limited onboard computational resources is still an open challenge. In recent years, neuromorphic electronics and computing have demonstrated their capabilities in building efficient and compact intelligent robotic systems capable of sensing and perception in real-world environments [39]. Neuromorphic computing aims to solve perceptual sensing and inference at the sensor level [40], which employs analog/digital signals collected from bioinspired sensors to implement neural computational primitives. These computational primitives are advantageous in processing context-dependent information at different time scales. In addition, event-driven sensors (e.g., tactile sensors and dynamic vision sensors) have become popular in scenarios with sparse activity, which can effectively reduce the transmission, storage, and processing of redundant data [41, 42].

7.5 Opportunities and Challenges of Hospital Automation Robotics

In Chap. 6, we summarized currently available applications for automation within the healthcare sector and envisioned potential solutions for smart hospitals in the future. With the richness of this research field, there still exist diverse opportunities and challenges for the development of hospital and automation robotics.

7.5.1 Multidisciplinary and Application-Centered Technologies

We must develop new application-oriented robots by integrating multidisciplinary technologies so that they can be easily adopted by different end users and in multiple clinical scenarios. The new generation of medical robots must be reliable, safe, and quickly deployable when needed. The main applications, as mentioned earlier, include hospital logistics, pharmacy and drug management, patient transfer and care, high throughput lab automation, and diagnosis and imaging. For hospital logistics and patient transfer and care, the opportunity lies in improved navigation within unmapped or cluttered environments. For example, autonomous robots should be able to continuously navigate and complete given tasks. Patient transfer and care robots should enhance clinical workflows in the key areas of a hospital, such as the ICU and general patient wards, and be able to interact directly with patients by measuring vital signs, key biomarkers, and delivering needed treatments. Similarly, this frees medical staff from time-consuming work and allows them to focus on their main tasks, such as patient treatment and care.

In order for specific robots to be accepted by healthcare workers, public safety officials, business owners, and individuals, the robots must be technologically mature. *National Aeronautics and Space Act* (NASA) assesses technology maturity through both the *Technology Readiness Level* (TRL) for the individual technology and the *Technology Readiness Assessment* (TRA) for the system maturity [43]. Commonly, low technology maturity challenges have led respondents to reject low TRL robots or high TRL robots with low TRA. As an emerging area, we have witnessed rapid development of hospital automation robots and a number of robotic systems with a low level of technical maturity serving as hospital-sanctioned experiments. The challenge lies in how to design reliability, safety, and safeguards from unintended consequences so that suitable solutions can be rapidly deployed and scaled for smart hospitals.

7.5.2 Improved Human–Robot Cooperation

The next-generation hospital automation robots need to better interact with end users. Improved sensor technology will empower robots to safely interact with their known/unknown environment, including objects, human workers, or other robots. This will require greater flexibility and deployment of the robot [44]. For remote operating systems or telepresence robots, flowless integration and high availability with operational workflows are critical for user acceptance, safety, and security. Remote robotic operation is already a mature technology in industry and medicine [45]. Specifically, advanced technologies, such as AR/VR, as well as high-speed wireless communication, could further improve the operation of telerobotics. Eventually, robots should be able to assist in surgeries, rehabilitation, or personal care by allowing remote treatment anywhere, anytime.

For infectious diseases, asymptomatic individuals can become potential carriers. Here, the opportunity lies in the development of ergonomics and application-specific haptic devices that allow users to sense the environment in which robots are deployed and make decisions accordingly. In terms of control strategies, we need to develop robotic systems with a higher level of autonomy. For example, clinicians can train robots to perform routine or complicated tasks, where imitation learning techniques can be used to teach the robots.

7.5.3 Increased Autonomy and Ethical Challenges

With the continuous growth of autonomous levels of hospital automation robots, the frequent interaction with medical staff and patients poses a series of ethical and safety challenges. Robots, especially when being operated in a healthcare environment, are data-driven, meaning they access sensitive patient information. It is therefore important to consider potential ethical and legal regulations [24]. Important concerns include privacy, ownership, data governance, and trust.

One ethical challenge is that robots used in patient transfer and care should be treated as ethical impact agents as they are highly related to human safety and health [46]. Ethical impact agents increase the professional obligation of the designer to ensure that the robot operates reliably and that users are aware of the implied consequences of use, including dangers and hidden costs. The second ethical challenge is protecting people and the environment. For example, robot-assisted disinfection in a random and long-term manner may expose patients and medical staff to health risks. The third ethical challenge is human rights and privacy, especially in healthcare applications. Unlike public safety, hospitals and public health agencies are less vulnerable because they often have institutional review boards that decide when and how to introduce new technology into their businesses. However, these decision-makers may not be aware of potential ethical consequences. It would be unethical for roboticists to shift the blame to the agency. It appears that robot manufacturers are donating equipment to encourage these institutions to carry out experiments and thus assume some ethical responsibility. Despite the many challenges mentioned above, one thing for certain is that the future of medical robotics is bright, and it is set to transform our healthcare system for many years to come.

7.6 Conclusions

Medical robotics for surgery, personalized rehabilitation, hospital automation, and high-throughput screening represents an important area of growth globally. As a clinical emphasis on improved surveillance and earlier diagnosis increases, medical robotics is moving toward precision intervention. This requires improved quality, minimally invasive access, and an unprecedented level of accuracy. There are many platforms available from both commercial and research organizations that are more agile and intelligent than early-generation medical robots. By solving the remaining open challenges, medical robotic systems offering improved safety, efficacy, and reduced costs will soon make them a mainstream clinical practice, and they will also define the future of smart hospitals and home-based patient care.

References

1. Dupont PE, Nelson BJ, Goldfarb M, et al. A decade retrospective of medical robotics research from 2010 to 2020. Sci Robot. 2021;6(60):eabi8017.
2. Troccaz J, Dagnino G, Yang G-Z. Frontiers of medical robotics: from concept to systems to clinical translation. Annu Rev Biomed Eng. 2019;21:193–218.
3. Yang G-Z, Bellingham J, Dupont PE, et al. The grand challenges of science robotics. Sci Robot. 2018;3(14):eaar7650.
4. Ciuti G, Valdastri P, Menciassi A, et al. Robotic magnetic steering and locomotion of capsule endoscope for diagnostic and surgical endoluminal procedures. Robotica. 2010;28(2):199–207.
5. Dogangil G, Davies B, Rodriguez Y, Baena F. A review of medical robotics for minimally invasive soft tissue surgery. Proc Inst Mech Eng H J Eng Med. 2010;224(5):653–79.
6. Cossetto T, Zareinia K, Sutherland G. Robotics for neurosurgery. In: Medical robotics. Oxford: Elsevier; 2012. p. 59–77.
7. Vitiello V, Lee S-L, Cundy TP, et al. Emerging robotic platforms for minimally invasive surgery. IEEE Rev Biomed Eng. 2012;6:111–26.
8. Kundrat D, Dagnino G, Kwok TM, et al. An MR-safe endovascular robotic platform: design, control, and ex-vivo evaluation. IEEE Trans Biomed Eng. 2021;68(10):3110–21.
9. Attanasio A, Scaglioni B, de Momi E, et al. Autonomy in surgical robotics. Ann Rev Control Robot Auton Syst. 2021;4:651–79.
10. Chang WH, Kim YH. Robot-assisted therapy in stroke rehabilitation. J Stroke. 2013;15(3):174–81.
11. Awad LN, Bae J, O'Donnell K, et al. A soft robotic exosuit improves walking in patients after stroke. Sci Transl Med. 2017;9(400):eaai9084.

12. Freivogel S, Mehrholz J, Husak-Sotomayor T, et al. Gait training with the newly developed 'LokoHelp'-system is feasible for non-ambulatory patients after stroke, spinal cord and brain injury. A feasibility study. Brain Inj. 2008;22(7–8):625–32.
13. Chase A. New assistive devices for stroke rehabilitation. Nat Rev Neurol. 2014;10(2):59.
14. Cheng N, Phua KS, Lai HS, et al. Brain-computer interface-based soft robotic glove rehabilitation for stroke. IEEE Trans Biomed Eng. 2020;67(12):3339–51.
15. Broekens J, Heerink M, Rosendal H. Assistive social robots in elderly care: a review. Geron. 2009;8(2):94–103.
16. Ktistakis IP, Bourbakis NG. Assistive intelligent robotic wheelchairs. IEEE Potentials. 2017;36(1):10–3.
17. Matarić MJ. Socially assistive robotics: human augmentation versus automation. Sci Robot. 2017;2(4):eaam5410.
18. Brose SW, Weber DJ, Salatin BA, et al. The role of assistive robotics in the lives of persons with disability. Am J Phys Med Rehabil. 2010;89(6):509–21.
19. Wu R, Wang J, Chen W, et al. Design of a transfer robot for the assistance of elderly and disabled. Adv Robot. 2021;35(3–4):194–204.
20. Bloss R. Mobile hospital robots cure numerous logistic needs. Ind Robot. 2011;38:567–71.
21. Kovach CR, Taneli Y, Neiman T, et al. Evaluation of an ultraviolet room disinfection protocol to decrease nursing home microbial burden, infection and hospitalization rates. BMC Infect Dis. 2017;17(1):1–8.
22. Gu E, Tang X, Langner S, et al. Robot-based high-throughput screening of antisolvents for lead halide perovskites. Joule. 2020;4(8):1806–22.
23. Greenaway R, Santolini V, Bennison M, et al. High-throughput discovery of organic cages and catenanes using computational screening fused with robotic synthesis. Nat Commun. 2018;9(1):1–11.
24. Yang G-Z, Cambias J, Cleary K, et al. Medical robotics—regulatory, ethical, and legal considerations for increasing levels of autonomy. Am Assoc Adv Sci. 2017;2:eaam8638.
25. Heng W, Solomon S, Gao W. Flexible electronics and devices as human–machine interfaces for medical robotics. Adv Mater. 2022;34(16):2107902.
26. Lin Z, Gao A, Ai X, et al. ARei: augmented-reality-assisted touchless teleoperated robot for endoluminal intervention. IEEE/ASME Trans Mechatron. 2021;27:3144–54.
27. Luo X, Mori K, Peters TM. Advanced endoscopic navigation: surgical big data, methodology, and applications. Annu Rev Biomed Eng. 2018;20:221–51.
28. Fu Z, Jin Z, Zhang C, et al. The future of endoscopic navigation: a review of advanced endoscopic vision technology. IEEE Access. 2021;9:41144–67.
29. Gulati S, Patel M, Emmanuel A, et al. The future of endoscopy: advances in endoscopic image innovations. Dig Endosc. 2020;32(4):512–22.
30. Subramanian V, Ragunath K. Advanced endoscopic imaging: a review of commercially available technologies. Clin Gastroenterol Hepatol. 2014;12(3):368–76.e1.
31. He Z, Wang P, Ye X. Novel endoscopic optical diagnostic technologies in medical trial research: recent advancements and future prospects. Biomed Eng Online. 2021;20(1):1–38.
32. Zhou X-Y, Guo Y, Shen M, et al. Application of artificial intelligence in surgery. Front Med. 2020;14(4):417–30.
33. Han J, Davids J, Ashrafian H, et al. A systematic review of robotic surgery: from supervised paradigms to fully autonomous robotic approaches. Int J Med Robot Comput Assist Surg. 2021;18:e2358.
34. Chi W, Dagnino G, Kwok TM, et al. Collaborative robot-assisted endovascular catheterization with generative adversarial imitation learning. In: Proceedings of the 2020 IEEE international conference on robotics and automation (ICRA). IEEE; 2020.
35. Saeidi H, Opfermann J, Kam M, et al. Autonomous robotic laparoscopic surgery for intestinal anastomosis. Sci Robot. 2022;7(62):eabj2908.
36. Xu W. Toward human-centered AI: a perspective from human-computer interaction. Interactions. 2019;26(4):42–6.

37. Rudovic O, Lee J, Dai M, et al. Personalized machine learning for robot perception of affect and engagement in autism therapy. Sci Robot. 2018;3(19):eaao6760.
38. Gunning D, Stefik M, Choi J, et al. XAI—explainable artificial intelligence. Sci Robot. 2019;4(37):eaay7120.
39. Bartolozzi C, Indiveri G, Donati E. Embodied neuromorphic intelligence. Nat Commun. 2022;13(1):1–14.
40. Indiveri G, Liu S-C. Memory and information processing in neuromorphic systems. Proc IEEE. 2015;103(8):1379–97.
41. Bartolozzi C, Ros PM, Diotalevi F, et al. Event-driven encoding of off-the-shelf tactile sensors for compression and latency optimisation for robotic skin. In: Proceedings of the 2017 IEEE/RSJ international conference on intelligent robots and systems (IROS). IEEE; 2017.
42. Scheerlinck C, Rebecq H, Gehrig D, et al. Fast image reconstruction with an event camera. In: Proceedings of the IEEE/CVF Winter Conference on Applications of Computer Vision. IEEE; 2020.
43. Hirshorn S, Jefferies S. Final report of the NASA Technology Readiness Assessment (TRA) study team. NASA Technology Readiness Assessment; 2016.
44. Feil-Seifer D, Haring KS, Rossi S, et al. Where to next? The impact of COVID-19 on human-robot interaction research. New York: ACM; 2020.
45. Avgousti S, Christoforou EG, Panayides AS, et al. Medical telerobotic systems: current status and future trends. Biomed Eng Online. 2016;15(1):1–44.
46. Moor JH. The nature, importance, and difficulty of machine ethics. IEEE Intell Syst. 2006;21(4):18–21.

Index

Y. Guo et al., *Medical Robotics*, Innovative Medical Devices,
https://doi.org/10.1007/978-981-99-7317-0

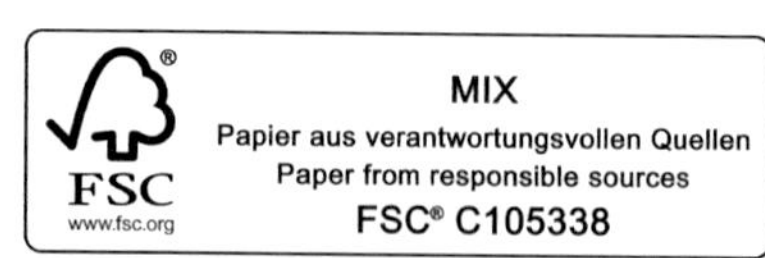

If you have any concerns about our products,
you can contact us on
ProductSafety@springernature.com

In case Publisher is established outside the EU,
the EU authorized representative is:
Springer Nature Customer Service Center GmbH
Europaplatz 3, 69115 Heidelberg, Germany

Printed by Libri Plureos GmbH
in Hamburg, Germany